THE COMPLETE MRCP

Data Interpretation Questions and Case Histories

MRCP Part 2

For Churchill Livingstone:

Publisher : Laurence Hunter
Project editor : Barbara Simmons
Copy editor : Alison Bowers
Project controller : Nancy Arnott
Design direction : Erik Bigland

THE COMPLETE MRCP

Data Interpretation Questions and Case Histories
MRCP Part 2

H L C Beynon BSc MRCP
Consultant Physician
Department of Rheumatology
Royal Free Hospital
London

J B van den Bogaerde MBChB PhD (Cantab) FCP(SA) MMed Int MRCP
Professor of Physiology
University of Pretoria
South Africa;
Reader in Physiology
St Mark's Hospital
Harrow

K A Davies MA MD FRCP
Senior Lecturer and Honorary Consultant
Department of Medicine
Imperial College School of Medicine at the Hammersmith Hospital
London

Foreword by

Mark J Walport MA PhD FRCP FRCPath
Professor of Medicine, Chairman of the Division of Medicine, Imperial College
School of Medicine and Hammersmith Hospital, London

SECOND EDITION

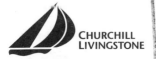

CHURCHILL
LIVINGSTONE

EDINBURGH LONDON NEW YORK PHILADELPHIA SAN FRANCISCO SYDNEY
TORONTO 1998

CHURCHILL LIVINGSTONE
An imprint of Harcourt Publishers Limited

© Longman Group Limited 1991
© Harcourt Brace and Company Limited 1998
© Harcourt Publishers Limited 2000

First edition 1991
Second edition 1998
 Reprinted 2000
 Reprinted 2001

ISBN 0 443 056943

British Library of Cataloguing in Publication Data
A catalogue record for this book is available from the British Library.

Library of Congress Cataloging in Publication Data
A catalog record for this book is available from the Library of Congress.

Medical knowledge is constantly changing. As information becomes available,
changes in treatment, procedures, equipment and the use of drugs become
necessary. The authors and publishers have, as far as it is possible, taken care to
ensure that the information given in this text is accurate and up to date.
However, readers are strongly advised to confirm that the information,
especially with regard to drug usage, complies with the latest legislation and
standards of practice.

Typesetting by IDS (India) Ltd
Printed in China

Foreword to The Complete MRCP

The MRCP examination aims to test a broad range of clinical skills and background knowledge at an early stage of training in general medicine. The Part 1 examination provides an assessment of general medical knowledge and the written Part 2 assesses the ability to interpret clinical data and to identify those physical signs that can readily be photographed.

The format of the examination is influenced by the large number of candidates and the necessity to provide a test of uniform standard. Multiple choice questions (MCQs) provide a standardised assessment of knowledge. Studies conducted in disciplines other than medicine have shown that MCQs provide a discriminator of abilities that correlates with other tests such as the writing of essays. Animated discussion of the answers to multiple choice questions posed in the examination often engenders paranoia about the ambiguity or idiocy of particular questions. In reality, the answers to clinical questions are rarely black and white, as demanded by MCQs. However, the occasional obscure or ambiguous question that slips into the exam will be detected during marking of the papers and will not be used again. Such questions will only damage individual candidates if the fury they engender at the time disturbs a balanced approach to answering the remainder of the questions. The 'grey' cases and photographic questions provide tests that approximate more closely to the reality of the bedside and probe comprehension of relevant clinical physiology and pathology.

This series of three books has been written by a team of physicians who have not yet forgotten the agonies of the MRCP examination and who participate actively in teaching others who are about to confront the same hurdle. These books provide stimulating examples of the types of question encountered in all three sections of the MRCP examination, and provide an entertaining and informative journey through many of the highways and byways of medicine

London 1998   M.J.W.

Preface

This is the second book in the series 'The Complete MRCP' and is complementary to books 1 and 3. Book 1 contains 300 MCQs with expanded answers and covers Part 1 of the MRCP. Book 3 covers the photographic interpretation section of Part 2 of the MRCP exam.

This book contains a collection of data interpretation questions and case histories similar to that encountered in Part 2 of the MRCP examination.

We hope this series will be both stimulating and helpful for candidates preparing for the examination.

1998

H.L. Beynon
J.B. van den Bogaerde
K.A. Davies

Table of normal values

Urea, electrolytes and liver function tests

Sodium	136–149 mmol/l
Potassium	3.8–5 mmol/l
Bicarbonate	24–30 mmol/l
Urea	2.5–6.5 mmol/l
Chloride	93–108 mmol/l
Creatinine	55–125 µmol/l
Total protein	65–80 g/l
Albumin	35–55 g/l
Calcium	2.15–2.65 mmol/l
Phosphate	0.80–1.4 mmol/l
Bilirubin	2–13 µmol/l
Alkaline phosphatase	30–130 iu/l
Aspartate amino-transferase	5–27 iu/l
Uric acid	0.1–0.4 mmol/l
Gamma GT	0–30 iu/l
Creatine kinase	0–170 iu/l
Plasma osmolality	285–295 mosmol/kg

Miscellaneous

Cholesterol	3.6–7.2 mmol/l
Triglyceride	0–1.5 mmol/l
Glucose	3.5–5.5 mmol/l
Immunoglobulins	
IgG	5–16 g/l
IgA	1.25–4.25 g/l
IgM	0.5–1.7 g/l
C-reactive protein	0–10 mg/l
Iron	
males	16–30 µmol/l
females	11–27 µmol/l
Total iron binding capacity	45–72 µmol/l
Vitamin B_{12}	200–900 pg/ml
Serum folate	1.8–14 µg/l
Magnesium	0.65–1 mmol/l
Faecal fat excretion	11–18 mmol/l

Hormone levels

Cortisol	
9 am	170–720 nmol/l
midnight	170–220 nmol/l
Growth hormone	<10 ng/ml
Thyroxine	70–160 nmol/l
Thyroid-stimulating hormone	0.8–3.6 mU/l

Haematology

Haemoglobin	
males	13.5–17.5 g/dl
females	11.5–15.5 g/dl
Red blood cell count	
males	$4.5–6.5 \times 10^{12}$/l
females	$3.9–5.6 \times 10^{12}$/l
Packed cell volume	
males	0.4–0.54 l/l
females	0.35–0.47 l/l
Mean corpuscular haemoglobin	27–32 pg
Mean corpuscular haemoglobin concentration	32–36 g/dl
Mean corpuscular volume	76–98 fl
Reticulocyte count	0.2–2%
Platelet count	$150–400 \times 10^{9}$/l
White blood count	$4–11 \times 10^{9}$/l
Neutrophils	$2.5–7.58 \times 10^{9}$/l
Lymphocytes	$1.5–3.5 \times 10^{9}$/l
Eosinophils	$0.04–0.44 \times 10^{9}$/l
Basophils	$0–0.1 \times 10^{9}$/l
Monocytes	$0.2–0.8 \times 10^{9}$/l
Erythrocyte sedimentation rate	0–10 mm in the first hour
Prothrombin time	12–15.5 sec
Activated partial thromboplastin time	30–46 sec
Thrombin time	15–19 sec
Bleeding time	2–8 mins
Fibrinogen	2–4 g/l

Cardiology normal values

	Mean (mmHg)	Range (mmHg)
R.A.	4	0–8
R.V.		
systolic	25	15–30
end diastolic	4	0–8
P.A.P.		
systolic	25	15–30
diastolic	10	5–15
mean	15	10–20
P.A.W.P.	10	5–14
L.V.		
systolic	120	90–140
end diastolic	7	4–12
Aorta		
systolic	120	90–140
diastolic	70	60–90
mean	85	70–105

Questions

1 A 60-year-old woman was brought to casualty unconscious. Her blood glucose was 2.6 mmol/l. She was resuscitated with intravenous glucose. She gave a 3-month history of early morning dizziness. Past medical history was unremarkable.

Investigations:

Fasting blood glucose	2.7 mmol/l
Blood insulin	16 mU/l
Hb	14 g/dl
MCV	84 fl

Urea/electrolytes/liver function tests normal

a) What is the diagnosis?
b) What is the differential diagnosis and how would you distinguish between them?

2 This patient presented with recurrent collapse. She was on no drugs.

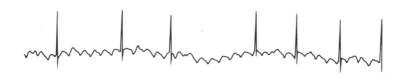

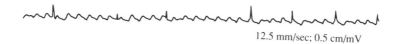

12.5 mm/sec; 0.5 cm/mV

a) What is the likely underlying disease?
b) What treatment will be required?
c) What is the theoretical danger of atrioversion with quinidine?

3 A 32-year-old non-smoker is admitted for investigation and treatment of severe shortness of breath. The following results are obtained:

Hb	14.3 g/dl
WCC	$15.4 \times 10^9/l$
Neutrophils	74%
Lymphocytes	12%
Eosinophils	11%
pO_2	8.4 kPa
pCO_2	5.4 kPa
PEFR	80 l/sec
Flow–volume loop	A

The patient's condition deteriorates over the next 12 hours and he is subsequently electively ventilated via a cuffed endotracheal tube. He is weaned from the ventilator 4 weeks later. A flow–volume loop is performed 4 months later (B).

a) What diagnosis would account for i) the first and ii) the second flow–volume loops?

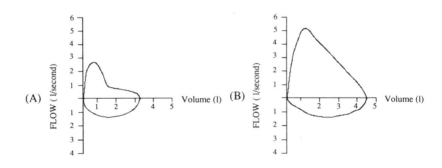

Question 4

4 A 10-year-old Asian girl attended hospital complaining of a 10-day history of fever and malaise. Her ankles, right wrist and left knee had been stiff and painful for 5 days. Her general practitioner had seen her 2 weeks previously and given her a course of antibiotics for a sore throat and mild upper respiratory tract infection. She was treated with aspirin, following which her fever settled over 48 hours and her joints became much less painful.

She had no previous history of joint problems. Twelve weeks before, she had returned from a 6-week holiday in Pakistan, where both she and her brother had contracted hepatitis. She had received primary chemoprophylaxis for tuberculosis at the age of nine.

Examination

Temperature 39°C, no pharyngitis, no lymphadenopathy, no skin rashes. Pulse 90 regular, JVP not elevated, normal first and second heart sounds and a soft pericardial rub. She had no hepatosplenomegaly. The painful joints were swollen.

Investigations:

Hb	10 g/l
MCV	80 fl
WBC	12×10^9/l 70% neutrophils
Platelets	400×10^9/l
Haemoglobin electrophoresis	normal
Urea and electrolytes	normal
Bilirubin	7 μmol/l
Aspartate amino-transferase	65 iu/l
ESR	115 mm in the first hour
Latex and autoantibody screen	negative
IgG	25 g/l
IgA	3.14 g/l
IgM	2.11 g/l
C-reactive protein	80 mg/l
Cultures of blood, urine and throat	negative
Paul–Bunnell	negative
Hepatitis B Ag	negative
Hepatitis A antibodies – acute serum	1/1280
– convalescent serum 1/640	

ASO titre 500 iu/l acute serum, 800 iu/l convalescent
Left knee aspirate 20 ml of yellow fluid containing 3000 neutrophils/ml, sterile on culture
Urinalysis a trace of protein but no casts or cells on microscopy
CXR NAD, X-rays of the affected joints NAD
ECG sinus rhythm, PR interval 0.3 ms, normal axis, normal QRS
Echocardiogram — mild mitral regurgitation, small pericardial effusion

a) What is the most likely diagnosis?
b) What treatment would you give?

5 A A middle-aged woman was referred with thirst, polydipsia and polyuria. She had been involved in a road traffic accident 9 months before and thought her symptoms had begun soon after this. She had no serious illness in the past and took no medication. General examination was normal, BP 120/80 no postural drop. Her 24-hour urine collections were between 7 and 12 litres.

Investigations:

Sodium	130 mmol/l
Potassium	3.5 mmol/l
Urea	2.0 mmol/l
Glucose	5 mmol/l
Protein	70 g/l
Albumin	35 g/l
Alkaline phosphatase	80 iu/l
Bilirubin	5 μmol/l
Plasma osmolality	268 mOsmol/kg
Urine osmolality	50 mOsmol/kg

a) What is the likely diagnosis?
b) What investigation would you arrange?

B A 24-year-old army private was admitted with a 24-hour history of coughing up bright red blood, and haematuria. On examination he was slightly agitated, temperature 37.2°C, pulse 100 and regular. Chest was clear to auscultation.

Investigations:

Hb	13.6 g/dl
WBC	7×10^9/l
Platelets	278×10^9/l
ESR	8 mm in the first hour
Urea	4 mmol/l
Chest X-ray	normal
Urine dipstick	protein ++, blood +++
Urine microscopy	100 RBC per high powered field; numerous epithelial cells Gram-positive cocci, gram positive rods, fusiform bacilli

a) What one diagnostic test would you perform to confirm your diagnosis?

6 A A 65-year-old lady with disseminated carcinoma of the ovary is admitted for a further course of chemotherapy. Four days after admission she complains of perioral paraesthesia.

Investigations:

Sodium	137 mmol/l
Potassium	4 mmol/l
Bicarbonate	26 mmol/l
Urea	5 mmol/l
Creatinine	120 µmol/l
Calcium	1.6 mmol/l
Phosphate	1.20 mmol/l
Albumin	37 g/l
Alkaline phosphatase	110 iu/l

a) What two signs would you attempt to elicit?

b) What is the underlying biochemical abnormality, what is its origin and how should the patient be treated?

B A 65-year-old man is admitted through casualty with marked shortness of breath. On examination he is in atrial fibrillation with a radial rate of 145 and an apical–radial deficit of 30, blood pressure 148/92 mmHg, JVP elevated at 8 cm, cardiomegaly, gallop rhythm and an apical pansystolic murmur. Both lung bases are dull to percussion and there are end-inspiratory crepitations to the mid zones. Gross pitting ankle oedema to the mid thighs is present. On admission he is taking no regular medication.

Investigations:

Sodium	128 mmol/l
Potassium	2.9 mmol/l
Bicarbonate	30 mmol/l
Urea	8 mmol/l
Albumin	24 g/l
Bilirubin	43 µmol/l
Alkaline phosphatase	601 iu/l
Aspartate amino-transferase	40 iu/l
Chest X-ray	upper lobe blood diversion, alveolar oedema and bilateral effusions

a) What is the diagnosis?

b) How do you explain the biochemical abnormalities?

7 A 30-year-old car mechanic presented to a follow-up clinic with an 8-week history of night sweats sufficient to soak the sheets, and right upper quadrant pain. He has lost 6 kg in 3 months and was drinking 2 pints of beer daily. On examination he was pyrexial 38.3°C, thin and pale with four-fingers' breadth of tender hepatomegaly. He had no lymphadenopathy and was not icteric.

Past medical history: Hodgkin's disease stage III diagnosed 1 year previously, treated with combined chemotherapy.

Investigations:

Hb	11.8 g/dl
WBC	2.4×10^9/l — 70% neutrophils
Platelets	345×10^9/l
Sodium	139 mmol/l
Potassium	4.5 mmol/l
Bicarbonate	27 mmol/l
Creatinine	87 μmol/l
Alkaline phosphatase	372 iu/l
Aspartate transaminase	79 iu/l
Bilirubin	24 μmol/l
Albumin	36 g/l
Protein	72 g/l
CXR	diffuse bilateral infiltration with occasional nodules

a) List 3 possible causes of this clinical picture.
b) List 3 important diagnostic procedures.

8 An 11-year-old girl presents with a 4-hour history of passing fresh blood per rectum. Past medical history is unremarkable. Earlier that day she had played a 2-hour game of tennis. She is on no regular medication and there is no significant family history. On examination she has a regular pulse of 120 and a blood pressure of 100/65 mmHg supine and 80/55 mmHg erect. Oral mucosa is normal. The abdomen is soft and there is no organomegaly. Rectal examination and sigmoidoscopy reveal normal perianal skin and normal rectal mucosa.

Investigations:

Hb	12 g/dl
MCV	83 fl
WBC	5×10^9/l
Platelets	240×10^9/l
PT	12 s
PTTK	36 s
Urea and electrolytes	normal
Chest X-ray	normal

The patient is resuscitated. An emergency gastroscopy is performed which shows normal stomach and duodenum.
a) What is the likely diagnosis?
b) How would you confirm your diagnosis?

9 A 50-year-old man is admitted for investigation of recurrent peptic ulceration. His problems first started at 43 years of age when he was resident in Delhi and was admitted for emergency surgery to repair a perforated peptic ulcer. Three years later he underwent a Polya partial gastrectomy for recurrent peptic ulceration. Since this time he has been persistently troubled by abdominal pain, worse at night, and diarrhoea with 4 loose motions a day. His current medication is ranitidine 150 mg 12-hourly together with liberal doses of antacids.

Investigations:

Hb	10 g/dl
MCV	76 fl
MCH	26 pg
MCHC	30 g/dl
Urea and electrolytes	normal
Liver function tests	normal
Fasting serum gastrin	390 pmol/l
	(Normal <100 pmol/l)

Secretin test — intravenously 2 units GIH secretin per kg

Basal fasting	value	401 pmol/l
	10 min	265 pmol/l
	20 min	280 pmol/l
	30 min	300 pmol/l

a) What is the diagnosis?
b) How would you confirm your diagnosis?

10 A 40-year-old Chinese man, who was otherwise fit and well, was admitted for a hernia repair. He had lived and worked in the UK for 25 years. He drank no alcohol and took no herbal remedies or other medications. He had no history of illness in the past and had never had a blood transfusion. The following blood results were obtained:

Sodium	140 mmol/l
Potassium	4.0 mmol/l
Urea	6 mmol/l
Albumin	40 mg/l
AST	120 iu/l
ALP	140 iu/l
Bilirubin	10 μmol/l
HBs Ag	negative
HBe Ag	positive
ANA	negative
Latex	negative

a) What is the likely diagnosis?
b) What further investigations does this man require?
c) What are the indications for treatment of this condition?

11 A 77-year-old man presented to outpatients complaining of weakness in both legs. Over the previous 3 months he had felt listless and had lost 5 kg in weight. He had suffered from lumbar spondylosis for several years; 4 months ago he developed upper and mid back pain which had recently radiated round to his umbilicus and required regular codeine phosphate. Two weeks previously he had developed a mild fever and night sweats and had been given a short course of antibiotics. On direct questioning he admitted that recently his bowel habit had changed and he had needed regular glycerol suppositories. He smoked 20 cigarettes per day and suffered from chronic bronchitis with frequent infective exacerbations. Medication included salbutamol inhaler, and oral aminophylline.

On examination the patient was cachectic, alert and orientated. Temperature 38°C. There was no lymphadenopathy, clubbing, anaemia or jaundice. Examination of his chest revealed a mild expiratory wheeze in both lung fields. Cardiovascular examination was normal. His cervical spine was normal, the lower 6 thoracic and all lumbar vertebrae were tender. The cranial nerves and fundi were normal. Hip and knee flexion was weak bilaterally; other muscle groups had normal strength. Light touch and pinprick were reduced in both lower limbs with a sensory level just below the umbilicus. Vibration sense and proprioception were reduced in both feet. The tendon reflexes were present and equal. The plantar reflexes were extensor on both sides. Rectal tone was normal, voluntary contraction intact, the prostate gland was smooth with a normal sulcus.

Investigations:

Hb	14 g/l
WBC	8×10^9/l
Platelets	450×10^9/l
ESR	17 mm in the first hour
Sodium	140 mmol/l
Potassium	4 mmol/l
Urea	6.5 mmol/l
CRP	10 mg/l
Aspartate amino-transferase	27 iu/l
Alkaline phosphatase	170 iu/l
Creatine phosphokinase	20 iu/l
Acid phosphatase	0.8 u/l (normal <3.3 u/l)

CXR lung fields clear, the 8th and 9th thoracic vertebrae were sclerotic and reduced in height; there was loss of the intervertebral disc space.
ECG sinus rhythm 76, normal axis.

a) What is the most likely diagnosis?
b) What investigations would you request and what treatment would you advise?

12 A 12-year-old boy is referred to outpatients with nocturnal enuresis. His mother comments that he is easily tired by sport and is not doing well at school. He is normotensive and on the 8th centile for height.

Investigations:

Sodium	145 mmol/l
Potassium	2.8 mmol/l
Bicarbonate	35 mmol/l
Chloride	80 mmol/l
Urea	5 mmol/l
Glucose	4.4 mmol/l
24-hour urine	60 mmol of potassium
	60 mmol of sodium

a) What is the likely diagnosis?

13 A 35-year-old man is sectioned and admitted to the psychiatric ward with a diagnosis of acute schizophrenia. Six days later he becomes pyrexial and is unable to eat; his condition deteriorates over the next 24 hours and he becomes increasingly confused. On examination, positive findings are a temperature of 39.5°C, pulse of 130, blood pressure 145/90 mmHg, marked neck stiffness, normal fundi and symmetrically increased tone in all four limbs with flexor plantars.

Investigations:

Sodium	140 mmol/l
Potassium	4 mmol/l
Bicarbonate	28 mmol/l
Urea	5 mmol/l
Bilirubin	23 μmol/l
Alkaline phosphatase	120 iu/l
Aspartate amino-transferase	54 iu/l
Calcium	2.4 mmol/l
Creatinine kinase	980 iu/l
Glucose	4.3 mmol/l
Hb	12 g/dl
WBC	12×10^9/l
Platelets	230×10^9/l
Chest X-ray	normal
CT head	normal
CSF	
opening pressure	15 cm H_2O
cell count	3 lymphocytes/mm^3
protein	0.5 g/l
glucose	3 mmol/l
Blood cultures	sterile
Urine dipstiok	negative blood,
	negative protein

a) What is the likely diagnosis?

14 A 44-year-old man is admitted with a history of vomiting. He has been treated in the past for peptic ulceration and depression. He looks unwell, investigations show:

Hb	16.3 g/dl
WBC	$11.1 \times 10^9/l$
Platelets	$354 \times 10^9/l$
Sodium	138 mmol/l
Potassium	2.8 mmol/l
Urea	14.3 mmol/l
pH	7.52
pO_2	12.4 kPa
pCO_2	5.5 kPa
Bicarbonate	36 mmol/l
Chloride	75 mmol/l

a) What is the metabolic abnormality?
b) What is the likely diagnosis?
c) Would the patient's urine be acid or alkaline?
d) Explain the basis of the metabolic upset in this situation.

15 A 25-year-old woman becomes unwell with fever, sore throat and dysphagia. On examination she has a temperature of 38°C, a fine tremor and a diffusely tender thyroid gland.

Investigations:

Hb	14 g/dl
WBC	$6 \times 10^9/l$
ESR	65 mm in the first hour
T4	190 nmol/l
^{99}Tc-isotope scan	no uptake

a) What is the diagnosis?
b) How would you treat her?

16 A 69-year-old man presents to his GP with a 4-month history of progressive weakness, and difficulty with swallowing and mastication. Examination reveals widespread wasting and fasciculation in upper and lower limbs, a wasted fasciculating tongue and a left partial ptosis.

a) Name two possible diagnoses, in order of likelihood.
b) Which finding makes one diagnosis more likely?
c) What investigations would you perform to distinguish these two possibilities?

17 A 56-year-old doctor returned to the UK after a 5-week holiday in Malaysia. He had an unremarkable past medical history and had been well up until 18 months previously when he started to complain of general lethargy. Over the past 4 months he lost 4.5 kg in weight and had developed low backache and intermittent diarrhoea. On average he smoked 25 cigarettes and drank 3 pints of beer each day. On examination he was suntanned, clinically anaemic and had several small nodes palpable in the axillae. Abdominal examination was normal. He was weak proximally but all reflexes were present and symmetrical. Mild pitting oedema was present.

Investigations:

Hb	10 g/dl
MCV	101 fl
MCHC	32 g/dl
WBC	$5 \times 10^9/l$
Platelets	$260 \times 10^9/l$
Urea	4 mmol/l
Creatinine	105 µmol/l
Sodium	135 mmol/l
Potassium	3.8 mmol/l
Albumin	28 g/l
Calcium	1.8 mmol/l
Phosphate	0.7 mmol/l
Alkaline phosphatase	188 iu/l
Bilirubin	17 µmol/l
Aspartate amino-transferase	25 iu/l
Faecal fat excretion	>26 mmol/l

a) What is the most likely diagnosis? How do you explain the neurological signs present?
b) How would you confirm your diagnosis?
c) What treatment would you institute?

18 This is the M-mode echocardiogram of a 17-year-old boy who faints with exercise.

a) Comment on structures A and B.

b) What is the pathophysiological significance of space C, and how will it be affected by squatting?

c) Give two reasons for the exertional syncope.

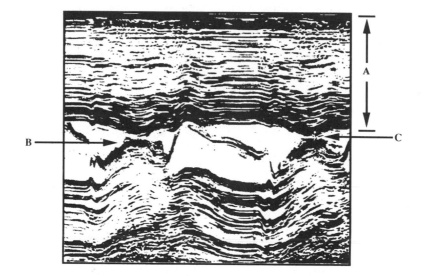

19 A 38-year-old lorry driver was referred with a rash presumed to be secondary to amoxycillin. He had presented to his GP 5 days before with a 6-day history of anorexia, fever and headache, and a 3-day history of dry cough and mild dyspnoea. He had no chest pain or haemoptysis. He smoked 10 cigarettes per day and drank 3–4 pints of beer per day. He had had no serious illness in the past. He had been commenced on amoxycillin 500 mg 8-hourly.

Examination: temperature 39°C, pulse 90, blood pressure 110/60. There was no clinical jaundice, anaemia, cyanosis or clubbing. Several fine crepitations could be heard in the right base. Over his trunk and upper arms he had a fine maculopapular rash; several target lesions were present. Otherwise general examination was normal. He was admitted to hospital.

Investigations:

Hb	13 g/dl
WBC	10×10^9/l
Sodium	142 mmol/l
Potassium	4.4 mmol/l
Urea	9 mmol/l
Creatinine	90 µmol/l
ESR	70 mm in the first hour
Aspartate transaminase	90 iu/l
Alkaline phosphatase	150 iu/l
Bilirubin	12 µmol/l
Blood and sputum culture	negative
Cold agglutinins	positive
CXR	patchy consolidation right base.

Five days after admission the patient developed increasing fatigue, dyspnoea, palpitations, dull central chest pain and myalgia.

Examination: pulse 120, blood pressure 110/60. Chest signs unchanged. Heart sounds: first and second sounds normal plus a soft third heart sound.

Blood gases	pO_2 14 kPa, pCO_2 5 kPa
CXR	no change
ECG	sinus tachycardia, widespread T-wave flattening and inversion.

Echocardiography showed normal valves and chambers. Contraction of the left ventricle was reduced.

a) Suggest a unifying diagnosis.
b) What further investigations would you arrange?

20 An 18-year-old man, previously fit and on no medication, becomes unwell with fever, myalgia, mild neck stiffness and loss of appetite. His GP diagnoses influenza. On review 48 hours later he is concerned that the patient is now clinically jaundiced and refers him to casualty.

Investigations:

Hb	14.8 g/dl
MCV	88 fl
Reticulocytes	1%
WBC	6×10^9/l
Platelets	259×10^9/l
ESR	10 mm in the first hour
Bilirubin	55 µmol/l
Conjugated bilirubin	9 µmol/l
Aspartate amino-transferase	25 iu/l
Alkaline phosphatase	105 iu/l
Albumin	42 g/l
Urea and electrolytes	normal

a) What is the likely diagnosis?

21 A 42-year-old epileptic is admitted through casualty having been found unconscious at home. The following results are obtained 24 hours later:

Sodium	135 mmol/l
Potassium	6.7 mmol/l
Urea	18 mmol/l
Creatinine	630 µmol/l
Calcium	1.84 mmol/l
Aspartate amino-transferase	86 iu/l
Gamma-glutamyl transpeptidase	70 iu/l
Urine dipstick	blood ++
Ammonium sulphate test	coloured supernatant
Red cell transketolase	low

a) What condition do these results suggest?
b) Suggest two possible causes in this patient.

22 The following results are obtained in a 32-year-old woman with a blood pressure of 184/114 mmHg.

Investigations:

Sodium	135 mmol/l
Potassium	5.2 mmol/l
Urea	11.2 mmol/l
Creatinine	212 μmol/l
Albumin	30 g/l
Urinalysis	Blood non-haemolysed trace
	Protein 5.4 g/24 h
Urine microscopy	Scanty red cells and granular casts
HbA1c	3.4%
ANA	1:320 speckled pattern
Renal biopsy	Immunofluorescence: Linear IgG on glomerular basement membrane

a) What is the diagnosis?
b) What histological pattern is likely to be present in the kidney?
c) What is the likely course of the disease?

23 A 65-year-old man is referred with glycosuria by his GP. He was asymptomatic, and on no regular medication. Six years ago he underwent surgery for a recurrent peptic ulcer.

A standard glucose tolerance test was performed.

Time	Blood glucose (venous) mmol/l	
0	4.8	No glycosuria
30 mins	12.5	
60 mins	9.8	Glycosuria
90 mins	2.3	
120 mins	3.2	

a) What does this investigation show?
b) What is the likely explanation in this case?

24 A 32-year-old woman presented with jaundice 2 months after starting the oral contraceptive pill and 1 month after returning from Turkey, where she had contracted a short-lived illness, characterized by fever and diarrhoea. She had felt run down for several months and attributed this to working long hours as a barmaid. In Turkey, while sunbathing, she had noticed several painless patches on her hands and face which did not tan. She was on no regular medication. She was a non-smoker and drank between 2 and 3 glasses of wine a day. On examination there were depigmented areas on both hands and on her face. She was icteric and several spider naevi were noted. Her heart, lungs and abdomen were normal.

Investigations:

Hb	12 g/l
WBC	8×10^9/l
Platelets	150×10^9/l
MCV	99 fl
Bilirubin	90 μmol/l
Aspartate amino-transferase	185 iu/l
Alkaline phosphatase	200 iu/l
Total protein	80 g/l
Albumin	26 g/l
HBS Ag	negative
Hep A serology	positive 1/640
Rheumatoid factor	negative
ANA positive	1/160

a) What is the most likely diagnosis?
b) What three investigations would you request?
c) What immediate management steps would you take?

25 A 30-year-old Asian man, born in Kenya and resident in the UK for 15 years, presented with an illness characterized by intermittent abdominal pain, fever and rigors. The illness had begun 3 weeks previously with diffuse colicky abdominal pains and night sweats. He had been prescribed antibiotics and was symptom free for 3 days. His symptoms then recurred accompanied by a dull frontal headache, muscle pains and severe fatigue. For the last week he had had a non-productive cough, anorexia and fevers up to 39°C accompanied by rigors and chills. He had no other abdominal or respiratory symptoms apart from the cough and abdominal pains. There was no relevant past medical history. He did not drink alcohol, smoke cigarettes or take any regular medication. He had no foreign travel apart from a holiday visiting his grandparents in Kenya 2 months before. He had obtained malaria prophylaxis before leaving the UK.

On examination his temperature was 39.8°C, pulse 110, BP 110/60 mmHg, respiratory rate 20/min. He was lethargic and when disturbed, belligerent. He had no jaundice, rash, lymphadenopathy or neck stiffness. Examination of his chest showed clear lung fields and a soft pansystolic murmur at the apex. There was diffuse abdominal tenderness predominantly in the upper quadrants. There was no abdominal guarding or rebound. Bowel sounds were normal but infrequent. PR examination was normal. A full neurological examination revealed no focal signs.

Investigations:

Haematology:
Hb 8.5 g/dl, MCV 87 fl, MCHC 30 pg, WBC $7 \times 10^9/l$ — 62% neutrophils, Platelets $128 \times 10^9/l$, ESR 80 mm in the first hour.

Biochemistry:
Glucose 6.2 mmol/l, Sodium 130 mmol/l, Potassium 4 mmol/l, Bicarb 20 mmol/l, Urea 30 mmol/l, Creatinine 495 μmol/l. Bilirubin 12 μmol/l, Alkaline phosphatase 50 iu/l, Aspartate amino-transferase 70 iu/l, Lactate dehydrogenase 495 iu/l, Amylase 60 iu/l, Creatinine kinase 50 iu/l, Albumin 28 g/l, Total protein 65 g/l, Calcium 1.7 mmol/l, Phosphate 1.19 mmol/l.

Miscellaneous:
Urine dipstick tests: blood +, protein +++
Urine microscopy: several granular and hyaline casts seen per high power field
Blood, throat, urine and sputum cultures all negative
Chest and abdominal X-rays normal
Abdominal ultrasound — normal kidneys, no gallstones, no lymph nodes
CT scan head normal
Lumbar puncture — clear CSF, 2 RBC and 3 WBC/mm³, Glucose 4.5 mmol/l, protein 0.3 g/l

a) What is the most likely diagnosis?
b) How would you confirm this?
c) What treatment would you give?

26 The patient has sustained an inferior myocardial infarction (ECG on facing page).

a) Which of the following drugs will exacerbate and which improve the problem demonstrated?

Digoxin	Verapamil
Isoprenaline	Adenosine
Atropine	Imipramine

27 You are performing a medical outreach clinic and are asked to see a 31-year-old staff nurse presenting with tiredness and symptoms of numbness and tingling affecting all fingers of the right hand. The pain is intermittent, but is most troublesome in the mornings. She has noticed a facial rash, associated with localised hyperpigmentation.

General examination is unremarkable, with a blood pressure of 105/70, pulse of 76 beats per minute. Axial and appendicular skeletal examination is normal. Tinel's sign is positive on the right side.

The available investigations show the following:

Sodium	132 mmol/l
Potassium	4.2 mmol/l
Urea	3.2 mmol/l
Creatinine	64 µmol/l

ALP 212 iu/l (normal <140 iu), AST 40 iu/l, Albumin 33 g/l, total protein 66 g/l, Hb 10.5 g/dl, normochromic normocytic; WCC 11.1 $\times$ 10^9/l, platelets 169 $\times$ 10^9/l. Complement levels: C3 120% of normal, C4 118% of normal human pool, CH50 17%.

a) What further investigations would you perform?

b) What other specific questions would you ask the patient in order to establish a diagnosis?

c) What is the likely explanation for the abnormal blood tests with which she presents?

d) Explain the complement test results.

28 A 16-year-old girl is reviewed 6-monthly, having been treated for acute lymphocytic leukaemia 10 years previously. She has recently returned from Greece where she has been living for the past 2 years. She presents with a 6-month history of weight loss of 8 kg, general malaise and occasional fevers. Clinical examination is normal apart from signs of obvious weight loss.

Full blood count, urea, electrolytes and liver function tests are all normal.

a) Give three possible diagnoses and your reasons.

b) How would you exclude two of these with further investigations?

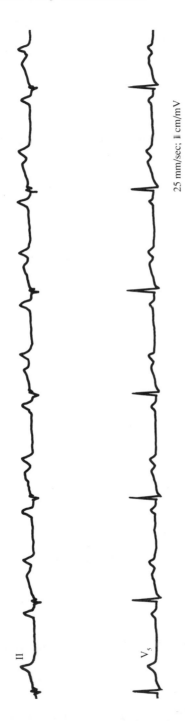

25 mm/sec; 1 cm/mV

II

V₅

29 A 55-year-old farmer complained of breathlessness and a dry cough which had worsened gradually over 3 months. Recently he had found working difficult because of dyspnoea and was considering retiring. He had occasional mild fevers and influenza-like symptoms and had lost 3 kg in weight over the past 2 months. Generally all of his symptoms were worse towards the end of the day. He had had an anterior myocardial infarct 5 years previously, complicated by left ventricular failure, now controlled with diuretics. He had had no further angina. He smoked 15 cigarettes daily until his myocardial infarction when on medical advice he had given up.

On examination there was no clubbing, anaemia, cyanosis, oedema or jaundice. The jugular venous pressure was normal, BP 150/70. Examination of his heart was unremarkable. On auscultation there were fine inspiratory crackles heard in both lung bases.

Investigations:

Hb	13.9 g/dl
WBC	10×10^9/l
ESR	50 mm in the first hour
Sodium	137 mmol/l
Potassium	3.9 mmol/l
Urea	8 mmol/l
Albumin	43 g/l
Total protein	78 g/l
Aspartate transaminase	35 iu/l
Alkaline phosphatase	111 iu/l
Bilirubin	12 μmol/l
Latex	negative
ANA	negative

ECG showed the previous anterior myocardial infarction, but was otherwise unremarkable. A chest X-ray showed areas of nodular shadowing in both lung bases.

FEV1 70%; FVC 80%, VA 110%, DLCO to 70%, KCO 60%.

Arterial oxygen saturation was 96% at rest and 92% on walking 100 metres.

a) What is the most likely diagnosis?

b) How would you confirm your diagnosis?

30 A The diagram below indicates the relationship of affected and unaffected members of a family with a rare enzyme defect.

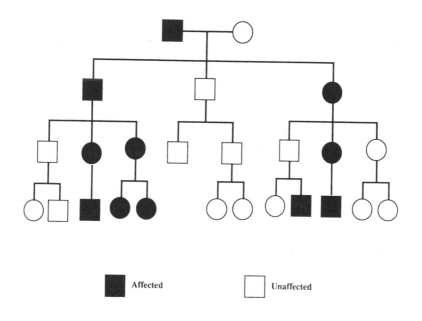

■ Affected   ☐ Unaffected

a) How is the condition inherited?
[Question continues overleaf]

B

a) In what Mendelian manner is this genetic trait transmitted?
b) Assuming penetrance is complete and that none of the family marries another carrier or affected individual, what is the risk of patients A, B, and C being affected? What would you estimate the risk to their children is?
c) List five important conditions transmitted in this way.

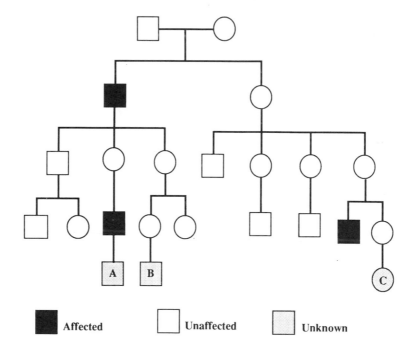

■ **Affected**   □ **Unaffected**   ▨ **Unknown**

31 A 44-year-old woman returns from Sri Lanka, having resided there for 5 years. Four months prior to leaving she developed an acute attack of gastroenteritis which settled initially. She then developed persistent colicky abdominal pain associated with loose bulky-stool diarrhoea and weight loss. She was investigated in Sri Lanka without success and was treated with oral metronidazole for presumed giardiasis. More recently she developed generalized aches and pains.

On examination she was clinically anaemic and pigmented. Abdominal examination was normal. Neurologically there was evidence of a proximal myopathy; in addition ankle jerks were absent and there was loss of vibration sense distally.

Investigations:

Hb	10.5 g/dl
MCV	108 fl
MCHC	32 g/dl
WBC	11×10^9/l
Albumin	29 g/l
Alkaline phosphatase	265 iu/l
Calcium	2.1 mmol/l
Phosphate	0.7 mmol/l
Aspartate amino-transferase	15 iu/l
Faecal fat	25 mmol/l
Stools	negative for ova cysts and parasites.

a) What is the most likely diagnosis?
b) Give a differential diagnosis.
c) How would you treat this patient?

32 A 70-year-old man presented with dull aching in both calves after moderate exercise. The symptoms had started 9 months earlier. Symptoms developed after walking 300–400 yards and settled after 5 minutes' rest, and would settle immediately if he sat down and stooped forward. Often, in addition to pain, he developed bilateral numbness in his thighs. He had no sphincter disturbance. He had had low back pain for many years. He had been depressed since his wife died. He smoked 20 cigarettes a day and was followed by a chest clinic for chronic obstructive airways disease. Medication included paracetamol as required, lofepramine 70 mg daily and two puffs from a salbutamol inhaler six-hourly.

On examination there was no rash, lymphadenopathy, clubbing, cyanosis or anaemia. His chest was clear, the heart sounds were normal, and the abdomen soft with no abnormal masses palpable. On inspection there was loss of his lumbar lordosis and reduced flexion and extension of the lumbar spine. Neurological examination of the cranial nerves and the upper limbs was normal. In the lower limbs tone power and coordination were normal; the reflexes were symmetrical but reduced compared to the upper limbs. The plantar reflexes were flexor. Soft touch and pin prick sensation were reduced from below the groin to just above the knees laterally. Proprioception and vibration sense were normal. The femoral, popliteal, posterior tibial and dorsalis anterior arterial pulses were present both at rest and after exercise.

Investigations:

Hb	14 g/dl
WBC	7.5×10^9/l
Platelets	455×10^9/l
Sodium	141 mmol/l
Potassium	3.9 mmol/l
Urea	7 mmol/l
Albumin	40 g/l
Calcium	2.3 mmol/l
Bilirubin	8 μmol/l
Aspartate transaminase	29 iu/l
Alkaline phosphatase	90 iu/l
IgG	15.5 g/l
IgA	2.2 g/l
IgM	3.0 g/l
Protein electrophoresis	normal
Bence–Jones protein	negative
CXR	consistent with mild obstructive airways disease
Lumbar spine X-ray	lumbar spondylosis with marked osteophyte formation

a) What is the most likely diagnosis?
b) What investigation might be done to confirm this diagnosis?

33 This M-mode echocardiogram is taken across the mid left ventricle. A is the left ventricular cavity and B is the interventricular septum.

a) What is abnormal about space A?
b) What is abnormal about space C?
c) Give two clinical signs that may be associated with space C.

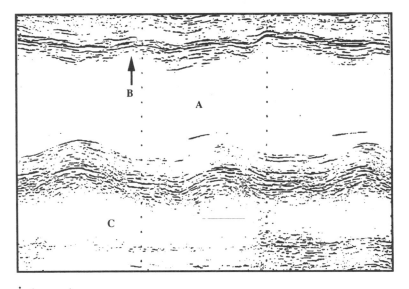

1 cm marker

34 A 32-year-old air-hostess presented with a 1-week history of fever and a migratory polyarthritis. For the last 2 days her left ankle and both knees had been painful and swollen but the other joints had settled. She had also developed tenosynovitis affecting the dorsum of her left hand. She was taking the oral contraceptive pill only. On direct questioning she had no other cardiorespiratory, abdominal, genitourinary or neurological symptoms.

On examination she had a hot swollen left ankle and left knee. Her right knee was tender only. In addition she had several vesicopustular lesions on her trunk, arms and lower legs.

Investigations:

Hb	14.5 g/dl
WBC	12 × 10⁹/l
Urea and electrolytes	normal
Rheumatoid factor	negative
Antinuclear factor	negative
Synovial aspiration	turbid fluid containing 35 000 neutrophils/ml
Blood cultures	negative
Synovial fluid	negative

a) What is the diagnosis?
b) How would you confirm your diagnosis?

35 A 25-year-old woman becomes profoundly unwell with diarrhoea and is brought to casualty.

On examination she is drowsy, neck stiffness is absent and no focal neurological signs are detected. Temperature 39°C, heart rate 110, blood pressure 70/20 mmHg. Marked bilateral conjunctivitis, and a widespread macular rash are apparent.

Investigations:

Hb	14.5 g/dl
WBC	14 × 10⁹/l
Platelets	100 × 10⁹/l
Urea	10 mmol/l
Creatinine	158 µmol/l
Potassium	5 mmol/l
Creatinine phosphokinase	400 u/l

a) What is the likely diagnosis?
b) How would you confirm your diagnosis?
c) How would you treat the patient?

36 A A 45-year-old woman undergoing treatment for depression was admitted to hospital. She was drowsy and had a marked tremor. ECG on admission showed flat T-waves.

Investigations:

Sodium	148 mmol/l
Potassium	4 mmol/l
Urea	14 mmol/l
T4	59 nmol/l
TSH	12 mU/l

a) What is the likely diagnosis?

B

a) What is the likely cause of this patient's coma?
b) Explain the abnormal investigations.

Sodium	114 mmol/l
Potassium	4.1 mmol/l
Urea	2.8 mmol/l
Creatinine	106 µmol/l
Aspartate amino-transferase	138 iu/l
Hb	11 g/dl
MCV	104 fl
WBC	5×10^9/l
Platelets	42×10^9/l
Cholesterol	6.4 mmol/l
Triglyceride	3.4 mmol/l

37 A 20-year-old girl presented to outpatients complaining of recurrent generalized itching and shortness of breath. In recent months she had had three episodes of pleurisy and mild shortness of breath on exertion. Her friends had commented to her that her holiday tan had lasted well into the winter. In the past she had experienced mild Raynaud's phenomenon which had required no treatment. She worked in an office and was not exposed to industrial dusts or chemicals. She took no regular medication and was a non-smoker. Her two maternal aunts had rheumatoid arthritis.

Examination revealed a fit-looking young woman who was well tanned. The skin on her forearms and fingers was boggy and oedematous but there was no desquamation. She had no lymphadenopathy, cyanosis, anaemia, clubbing or clinical jaundice. Her pulse was 80 regular, BP 150/90 mmHg, the jugular venous pressure was visible 1 cm above the angle of Louis. Her heart sounds were normal and there were several fine bilateral crackles heard at both lung bases.

Investigations:

Hb	13 g/dl
ESR	20 mm in first hour
CRP	10 mg/l
Urea	4.6 mmol/l
Creatinine	145 µmol/l
Rheumatoid factor	negative
Antinuclear antibody	1/80 homogeneous
Complement profile	normal
Serum angiotensin-converting enzyme	normal
Chest X-ray	bilateral fine linear shadowing/atelectasis
Ventilation/perfusion scan	normal
Lung function tests:	
FEV1	2.0 l
VC	2.4 l
PEFR	5.5 l/s
TLC	3.0 l
TLCO	80% predicted (80%)
VA	1.8 l (70%)
KCO	90% predicted

a) What is the most likely diagnosis?
b) What complications have occurred?

38 A 35-year-old woman was seen in casualty with a perianal abscess. On direct questioning she had had a number of episodes of diarrhoea in the past 2–3 years which had been treated by her doctor with loperamide and courses of antibiotics (including metronidazole). At the age of 9 months she had had pneumonia, which was followed throughout her childhood by numerous chest infections and occasional crops of boils. She thought that her family was generally subject to boils and attributed this to a poor diet, since her father had been unemployed. Her only other complaint was 'rheumatics' — she had a long history of joint pains and occasional joint swellings, affecting mostly the large peripheral joints and the wrists, but not the small joints in her hands or feet. Her only medication was Nuseals-aspirin as required for her joint symptoms.

Examination showed a cheerful but thin lady with no clubbing, anaemia or lymphadenopathy. Examination of her joints revealed mild crepitus in both knees and limited rotation and extension of both hips. Her neck and lumbar spine were normal for her age. The cardiovascular system and CNS were normal. Her spleen was just palpable. Rectal examination confirmed a perianal abscess.

Investigations:

Hb	12 g/dl
WBC	$4.0 \times 10^9/l$ — 55% neutrophils, 40% lymphocytes
Platelets	$200 \times 10^9/l$
ESR	15 mm in the first hour
Sodium	135 mmol/l
Potassium	4.0 mmol/l
Urea	5.0 mmol/l
Creatinine	130 μmol/l
Albumin	43 g/l
Total protein	60 g/l
Aspartate amino-transferase	20 iu/l
Alkaline phosphatase	90 iu/l
Bilirubin	6 μmol/l
Rheumatoid factor and ANA	negative
Cultures of blood and stool	negative
Culture of the abscess	S. faecalis
Chest X-ray	normal
X-rays of knees and hips	early osteoarthritis
Abdominal ultrasound	splenomegaly

a) What is the diagnosis?
b) What investigation would you request?
c) What treatments are of value?

39 A 27-year-old woman presents with a 2-day history of bleeding gums. On examination there are subconjunctival haemorrhages and patches of purpura.

Investigations:

Hb	6.4 g/dl
WBC	$32.5 \times 10^9/l$
Platelets	$32 \times 10^9/l$
Prothrombin time	20 s
APPT	50 s
Thrombin time	38 s
Fibrinogen	0.5 g/l

Film: numerous hypergranular promyelocytes present.

a) What is the likely diagnosis?
b) How would you confirm this diagnosis?

40 A A 50-year-old man complains of exertional dyspnoea. The following lung function results are obtained:
FEV 23%, VC 56%, FEV/VC 33% (40%), TLCO 69%, KCO 73%, VA 96%

a) Name two other useful pulmonary function tests.
b) What is the most probable diagnosis?

B The following lung function tests were obtained in a 55-year-old woman who was treated 10 years ago for an adenocarcinoma of the right main bronchus. She has remained well since then and is a non-smoker.
FEV 49%, VC 52%, FEV/VC 83% (98%), DLCO 75%, KCO 150%, VA 50%

a) How was her lung tumour treated?

C A 65-year-old man has a history of bony tuberculosis as a young man, resulting in gibbus deformity of the thoracic spine. He is admitted to hospital with increasing breathlessness and confusion. Admission blood gases are as follows:
pH 7.41, pCO_2 8.9 kPa, pO_2 6.1 kPa, Bicarbonate 42 mmol/l.

a) What is his respiratory problem?
b) What is the acid–base disturbance?

41 A 16-year-old boy is brought into A&E with a short history of severe headache and vomiting. He has a widespread maculopapular rash all over his body, and is very drowsy. He is staying with relatives away from home, and his parents are abroad. His uncle thinks that he may have been admitted to hospital on two previous occasions with similar problems, but does not know any details. The patient is too unwell to give a coherent history.

a) What other signs should be sought?
b) What initial investigations are required? How would the results influence your management? What is the probable diagnosis?
c) What therapy would you initiate in this patient? What complications may occur in this condition?
d) What other tests are required at a later date? What underlying problem needs to be considered in this patient?

42 A 32-year-old man presents with uncomfortable 'gritty' eyes, and painful knees — particularly on weight-bearing. He has just returned from a business trip to Bangkok.

a) What other questions would you ask when taking an initial history from this man?
b) What is the probable diagnosis? What important differential should be considered?
c) What other signs should be sought?
d) What other factors predispose to this condition?

43 A 39-year-old publican presents with a 6-month history of headache and malaise. He smokes 20 cigarettes a day, drinks regularly throughout the day and is on a thiazide diuretic for the treatment of mild hypertension.

On examination he is plethoric and hypertensive, blood pressure 190/115 mmHg. He has 3 cm hepatomegaly and 4 cm splenomegaly.

Investigations:

Hb	20.9 g/dl
WBC	14.9×10^9/l
Platelets	517×10^9/l
Sodium	143 mmol/l
Potassium	4 mmol/l
Urea	4.3 mmol/l
Bilirubin	24 µmol/l
Aspartate trans-aminase	63 iu/l
Alkaline phosphatase	163 iu/l
Uric acid	0.6 mmol/l
PO_2	12.8 kPa
pCO_2	5.3 kPa
PH	7.42

a) What is the likely diagnosis?
b) What further investigations are appropriate?

44 This 13-year-old underwent cardiac catheterization. Her parents had noticed that she was becoming increasingly breathless and blue.

	SAT O$_2$(%)	PRESS (mmHg)
RA	74	26 Mean
RV	76	110/5–10
PA	76	110/30
LV	92	105/0–10
Aorta	99	120/75

a) What waveform do you expect in the right atrial pressure trace and why?
b) Is the pulmonary valve functioning normally?
c) Describe any changes that you would expect between the vascular markings on the chest X-rays at 1 year and now.

45 You are asked to see a 69-year-old Hepatitis B-positive Asian man on the ward who has been receiving chemotherapy for peritoneal tuberculosis. He has become increasingly weak and his urine output has decreased dramatically over the previous week. He has a temperature of 38.4°C, and is complaining of pains in his wrists and elbows. His serum creatinine is 456 μmol/l, urea 23.1 mmol/l and potassium 2.4 mmol/l. Urinalysis shows + RBC, ++WBC, and + protein.

a) What further information should be obtained in the history?
b) What is the likely diagnosis? Why?
c) What other blood tests are required?
d) What other investigations are needed, and what findings would you expect?
e) What therapy is needed? Assuming that the patient requires renal replacement therapy acutely, what factors in the history may be relevant?

46 This patient has had recurrent syncope and heart failure.

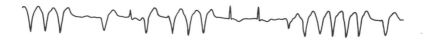

12.5 mm/sec; 0.5 cm/mV

a) What is demonstrated?
b) If there is nothing different on the 24-hour tape what difference in prognosis would be achieved by abolishing the arrhythmia pharmacologically?

47 A 57-year-old obese man is referred to outpatients with a history of visual disturbance. On two occasions he described transient loss of vision in the left eye. This came on over a few seconds, gradually obscuring all vision in that eye. After 3 or 4 minutes the vision cleared completely. On one occasion during an attack he was at his desk writing with his right hand, and noticed that his handwriting seemed to deteriorate, and he had difficulty holding his pen.

a) What is the likely diagnosis?
b) What other facts would you try to elicit in the history?
c) What physical signs should be sought?
d) How would you manage this patient?
e) What is the commonest cause of death in these patients?

48 A 37-year-old trout farmer presents with a 7-day history of fever, myalgias, nausea and severe frontal headache. He has experienced occasional colicky abdominal pain and vomited once. On two occasions he has noticed haematuria. One month previously he returned from his honeymoon in France but has not otherwise travelled abroad. At the age of 6 he suffered an episode of infectious hepatitis and there is a family history of diabetes mellitus. He drinks 5 pints of beer most evenings but does not smoke. He takes paracetamol occasionally for long-standing lower back pain.

On examination he is pyrexial 38.5°C and icteric. Bilateral subconjunctival haemorrhages and a purpuric rash over both calves are noted. There is no asterixis and he is alert. He has marked photophobia but no neck stiffness. In the abdomen he has smooth 4 cm hepatomegaly.

Investigations:

Hb	11.3 g/dl
WBC	15.9×10^9/l — 90% neutrophils
Platelets	470×10^9/l
Sodium	132 mmol/l
Potassium	4.5 mmol/l
Urea	27.8 mmol/l
Creatinine	305 µmol/l
Bilirubin	76 µmol/l
Aspartate amino-transferase	78 iu/l
Alkaline phosphatase	642 iu/l
PT	13 s
PTTK	32 s
Urine dipstick	protein++, blood++
Urine microscopy	occasional white cells, occasional red cells, no casts

a) What is the likely diagnosis?
b) How would you confirm your diagnosis?
c) What treatment would you recommend?

49 A 54-year-old man presents with a 4-hour history of severe, retrosternal chest pain and increasing shortness of breath. The pain started suddenly whilst eating, is constant in nature and radiates to the neck and interscapular region. In 1980 he was found to be hypertensive and is currently taking nifedipine slow release 20 mg 12-hourly. There is no other significant past medical history and no previous history of chest tightness. He smokes 20 cigarettes a day and drinks up to 6 pints of beer a day.

On examination he is distressed and clammy. Pulse 110 and regular, blood pressure 85/50 supine, JVP not elevated, heart sounds normal. All peripheral pulses are present and symmetrical. The left lung base is dull to percussion and breath sounds are decreased. Abdominal and neurological examination is normal. ECG shows sinus tachycardia and T-wave inversion in lead III. Chest X-ray shows a small left pleural effusion.

a) What is the diagnosis? Give a differential diagnosis.
b) How would you confirm your diagnosis?

50 A 45-year-old mentally subnormal woman presents in casualty with a broken arm after repeated falls. She has had epilepsy since childhood. Her last witnessed fit was 2 weeks ago; before this she had been fit-free for 2 years. Pulmonary tuberculosis had been diagnosed 6 months previously. Her medication consisted of phenytoin 400 mg, primidone 200 mg and Rifinah (combined rifampicin and isoniazid) 2 tablets daily.

Examination confirmed the fracture. In addition she had mild nystagmus and ataxia. Otherwise physical examination was normal.

Investigations:

Hb	11 g/l
MCV	105 fl
WBC	8×10^9/l — normal differential
Platelets	400×10^9/l
Sodium	136 mmol/l
Potassium	4.0 mmol/l
Urea	5 mmol/l
Albumin	40 g/l
Calcium	2.1 mmol/l
Phosphate	1.0 mmol/l
Bilirubin	6 μmol/l
Aspartate transaminase	28 iu/l
Alkaline phosphatase	180 iu/l

a) What is the diagnosis?
b) What investigations would you perform?

51 A A 29-year-old woman presents with progressive breathlessness on exertion, of 6 months' duration. Pulmonary function tests are performed:
FEV 90%, VC 92%, FEV/VC 96%, DLCO 59%, KCO 65%, VA 91%.
On exercise, arterial saturation measured by oximetry fell from 94% to 86% at 55% of predicted maximum workload.
a) Give two possible diagnoses.
b) Suggest two other relevant investigations.

B A 58-year-old man with rheumatoid arthritis complains of progressive breathlessness on exertion. On examination he is centrally cyanosed with fine crackles at both lung bases. Lung function results are as follows:
FEV 59%, VC 52%, FEV/VC 113%, TLC 80%, RV 77%, DLCO 23%, KCO 42%, VA 61%.
a) What is the most likely diagnosis?
b) Name two useful further investigations.

52 A 24-year-old man is brought into casualty in a semiconscious state after a football match on a Saturday afternoon. He smells strongly of drink.
a) What signs may be observed?
b) It seems likely that the patient is suffering from alcohol poisoning. What other possibilities must be considered?
c) What complications may ensue?
d) How would you treat this patient?

53 A 29-year-old woman presents to the clinic with a short history of headaches, which are worse in the morning, and double vision. On examination, the patient weighs 102 kg, there is papilloedema, and a partial right VI nerve palsy, but no other abnormal neurological signs.
a) What is the most likely diagnosis? Why? What other important possibility must be excluded?
b) What urgent investigation is required?
c) What is the main risk in this condition?
d) What is the treatment?

54 This patient is in casualty 2 hours after the onset of chest pain.
   a) Predict the appearance of the coronary arteriogram.
   b) What feature suggests that streptokinase has been given?
   c) What would be the significance of a period of atrioventricular nodal dissociation?
   d) What would you expect if the ECG has not changed in 1 year's time?

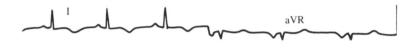

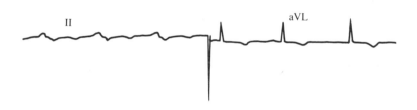

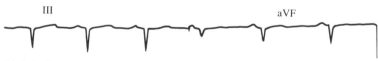

Limb leads

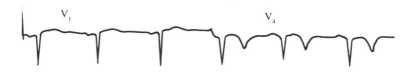

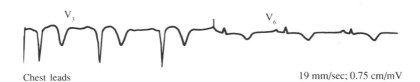

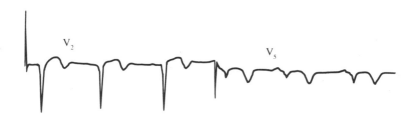

Chest leads

19 mm/sec; 0.75 cm/mV

55 This data was acquired from cardiac catheterization of a 26-year-old man with episodic dizziness.

	SAT O_2(%)	Press (mmHg)
RA	73	Mean 5
		A-wave 7
RV	75	97/0–10
PA	74	24/14
LV	96	130/0–10
Femoral artery	92	185/60

a) What is the most likely cause for the systemic desaturation?
b) What is the valve lesion?
c) Echocardiography shows a thick ventricular wall. What other abnormality do you suspect?
d) Give three possible causes for the dizzy spells.

56 A 34-year-old man presents with a 1-week history of pain in the left eye, associated with blurred vision. One year before, he had noticed that his ability to play tennis had been transiently impaired by apparent weakness of his right foot, but he had not sought medical advice as the symptoms had resolved after about a month. He had, however, been treated by his GP for acute labyrinthitis about 3 months before developing his current problem.

a) What is the likely diagnosis?
b) What signs might be elicited on examination of the eyes?
c) How would you interpret the patient's history prior to this acute presentation?
d) What investigations are required?
e) What is the prognosis of the ocular lesion? What will be the appearance of the optic disc 6 months later?

57 An 8-year-old boy is admitted following a grand mal convulsion. Routine blood investigations:

Glucose	4 mmol/l
Calcium	1.7 mmol/l
Albumin	39 g/l
Phosphate	1.9 mmol/l
Alkaline phosphatase	190 iu/l
Urea	4 mmol/l
Creatinine	75 μmol/l
Hb	11 g/dl

a) What is the cause of his convulsion?
b) Give a differential diagnosis and describe how you would investigate further.

58 This is data acquired at cardiac catheterization of a 32-year-old woman with dyspnoea.

	Sat O$_2$(%)	Press (mmHg)
RA	73	Mean 6
		A-wave 10
RV	74	60/0–10
PA	73	Mean 50
PACW		Mean 26 A-Wave 32
		End diastole 19
LV	98	120/0–10
Aorta	99	120/75

a) What is the primary lesion demonstrated?
b) Explain the high A-wave pressure in the right atrial measurement.
c) What may be palpated at the praecordium?
d) What is the underlying cardiac rhythm?

59 A 40-year-old man was admitted for investigation of an abnormal
chest X-ray which showed persistent linear shadowing and a
solitary nodular shadow in the left lower lobe. He had a dry
cough, occasional fever and had lost 4 kg in weight over a
3-month period. He smoked 20 cigarettes per day and drank
2–3 pints of beer per day. He worked in the construction industry
installing roofs. Recently he had been exposed to considerable
amounts of tile dust and in the past he had been exposed to
asbestos. One year before he had returned from a holiday pot-
holing in France and developed an acute illness characterized by
flitting arthralgia, a cough, left-sided chest pain, erythema
nodosum, fever and malaise. A chest X-ray was reported as
showing pneumonia and he received a course of penicillin and
then oxytetracyclin. However his symptoms settled slowly and he
was discharged home after 3 weeks.

On examination his temperature was 37.5°C, pulse 74 regular
and BP 110/70 mmHg. There was no palpable lymphadenopathy,
cyanosis, anaemia, jaundice or clubbing. Examination of the
chest revealed a normal heart and an area of dullness with
decreased breath sounds at the left lung base. Abdominal and
CNS examination were normal.

Investigations:

Hb	14 g/dl
WBC	11.8×10^9/l — neutrophils 85%
Platelets	400×10^9/l
Urea and electrolytes	normal
Glucose	5.3 mmol/l
Aspartate amino-transferase	28 iu/l
Alkaline phosphatase	130 iu/l
Bilirubin	6.0 µmol/l
Total protein	70 g/l
Albumin	30 g/l
Serum angiotensin-converting enzyme	normal
Tuberculin test	negative
Repeated blood cultures	negative
Lung function tests	within normal limits
ECG	normal

Chest X-ray: A single, well-defined, non-calcified nodule with
several linear shadows in the left lower lung field with marked
pleural thickening. There was no hilar lymph node enlargement.
Bronchoscopy: no endobronchial masses. Washings: no malignant
cells, macrophages+; culture negative for bacteria and tuberculosis.

An ultrasound-guided needle biopsy of the pleura and lung
tissue was obtained. Microscopic examination of the material
revealed no malignant cells and no acid-fast bacteria. There were
several necrotizing granulomas with multinucleated giant cells
and marked fibrosis.

a) What is the most likely diagnosis?
b) List three other important differential diagnoses.
c) Suggest two investigations.

60 A 26-year-old woman attends outpatients with a 2-month history of left hip pain — worse on weight-bearing and on exertion. Some relief is obtained from Ibuprofen. She has a complex previous medical history: 18 months previously she underwent a trans-sphenoidal hypophysectomy for a benign pituitary lesion which has resulted in pituitary failure. She had been on thyroid replacement therapy with 150 μg T4 for 2 years, and oestrogen therapy for 9 months. Perioperatively she had received 4 mg 6-hourly of dexamethasone for 3 weeks, and had been taking 2 mg 12-hourly for the last 12 months. Her weight was 102 kg; height 5ft 1 inch.

a) What is the most likely explanation for her hip pain? What other joints may be affected in this condition?
b) What investigations would you perform?
c) Was her endocrine replacement therapy entirely appropriate? Why might this be relevant?

61 A A 55-year-old man presents with a 12-hour history of severe abdominal pain and vomiting. He had been recently commenced on a thiazide diuretic for high blood pressure. On examination he was unwell, sweaty and tachycardic, with a blood pressure of 115/85 mmHg. His abdomen was diffusely tender and bowel sounds were absent.

Investigations:

Hb	13 g/dl
WBC	$14 \times 10^9/l$
Platelets	$245 \times 10^9/l$
Sodium	143 mmol/l
Potassium	3.9 mmol/l
Urea	9 mmol/l
Albumin	27 g/l
Calcium	1.9 mmol/l
Phosphate	0.8 mmol/l
Bilirubin	25 μmol/l
Aspartate transaminase	40 iu/l
Glucose	13 mmol/l
pO_2	8.8 kPa
pCO_2	4.0 kPa

a) What is the likely diagnosis and how would you confirm your diagnosis?
b) Suggest a possible cause in this case.

B A 49-year-old smoker is admitted to casualty having had a seizure at work. His colleagues describe a typical grand mal fit. The patient gives a further history of increasingly frequent severe headaches in recent months, and also difficulty in concentrating at work. His wife had noticed that he had been taking a good deal of time off, and seemed unusually cheerful and impulsive.

a) What is the probable diagnosis?
b) Which features in the history are important?
c) What investigations would you perform?

62 A 35-year-old woman is admitted confused, pyrexial and vomiting. Her flat-mate reports that she has been unwell for the last three months and has lost weight. Three days previously she was bed-bound with a severe cold. Her brother, who was called urgently by the flat-mate, collapsed in casualty, and was found to be hypoglycaemic. He responded to intravenous dextrose; it transpired that he missed his evening meal in his rush to visit his sister. He has been insulin-dependent for 5 years.

On examination the sister is disorientated in time and place, temperature 39°C, pulse 110 irregularly irregular with a blood pressure of 100/60. There is no neck stiffness and no focal neurological signs. The duty SHO has performed a lumbar puncture.

Investigations:

Hb	14 g/dl
WBC	$9 \times 10^9/l$ — 70% neutrophils
Sodium	140 mmol/l
Potassium	4 mmol/l
Urea	13 mmol/l
Albumin	35 g/l
Calcium	2.6 mmol/l
Phosphate	1.2 mmol/l
Glucose	5.2 mmol/l
CSF	Opening pressure 9 cm water
	Protein 0.6 g/l
	Glucose 4 mmol/l
	Cell count 3 lymphocytes/mm³

a) What is the likely diagnosis?
b) How would you treat the patient?

63 A 36-year-old West Indian male, who was a keen cricketer and opened the bowling for his local team, presented with acute pain and swelling in his right calf. A similar episode occurred in the winter 2 years previously. He was previously fit and well, but had a 2-year history of arthralgia affecting the small joints of both hands, and what he described as poor circulation in his feet.

Blood tests showed:
Hb 12.6 g/dl, WCC $9.3 \times 10^9/l$, with a normal differential, and platelets $97 \times 10^9/l$. Renal function tests were normal, total protein was 78 g/l with an albumin of 37 g/l. VDRL was positive.

a) What investigations would you perform: 1) blood tests, 2) radiological investigations?
b) What is the likely diagnosis, and what is the main differential?
c) What further investigations would be required?
d) How would you manage this patient?

64 A A 35-year-old woman is admitted to casualty with status epilepticus. The convulsion is terminated with diazepam. On recovering consciousness she gives a history of severe abdominal pain and vomiting and admits to having had two previous fits. She has noted progressive weakness in her right arm and is unable to grip a tennis racquet properly. On examination she looks well, is apyrexial with a regular pulse and blood pressure. There are no localizing signs in the abdomen. Neurologically there is a right radial nerve palsy — the rest of the examination is unremarkable.

Investigations:

Sodium	123 mmol/l
Potassium	4.0 mmol/l
Urea	4 mmol/l
Bilirubin	35 μmol/l
Aspartate transaminase	42 iu/l

a) Suggest a unifying diagnosis.
b) How would you confirm this diagnosis?

B A 3-week-old infant is seen with vomiting, diarrhoea and failure to thrive. On examination there is hepatomegaly and early cataracts are noted.

Blood glucose   1.9 mmol/l

a) What is the likely diagnosis?
b) What are the other recognized complications?
c) How would you confirm your diagnosis?
d) What treatment would you advocate?

Question 65

65 A 65-year-old woman was referred to outpatients with a 3-month history of progressive vertigo which was worse when she turned her head to the left. For 2 months she had had intermittent tinnitus and dull occipital headaches. General enquiry revealed that she had lost 4 kg of weight over 9 months, felt depressed and had lost her appetite. There was no relevant respiratory or cardiovascular history, no recent change in bowel habit and no genitourinary symptoms. She took bendrofluazide 2.5 mg daily and atenolol 50 mg daily for hypertension. In the past she had had an appendicectomy and a benign lump removed from her right breast. She was a lifelong non-smoker and consumed little alcohol.

Examination: weight 65 kg, temperature 37°C. There was no clubbing, cyanosis, jaundice or lymphadenopathy. There were no thyroid or breast masses. Pulse 60 regular, blood pressure 150/70 mmHg, heart and lungs normal. Examination of the abdomen revealed an appendicectomy scar only. She was well-orientated but had mild dysarthria and memory impairment. On walking she was clumsy and needed help to climb on to the couch; when walking in a straight line she tended to veer to the right. On right lateral gaze she had right beat nystagmus and several beats of rotatory nystagmus looking to the left. She had bilateral sensorineural deafness. Otherwise examination of the cranial nerves was normal. She had normal power and tone in all limbs. Both deep and superficial reflexes were symmetrical and normal. Coordination in her upper limbs was normal; there was no tremor and no dysdiadochokinesis. Sensation was normal.

Investigations:

Haematology
Hb 11 g/dl, MCV 84 fl, WBC 9.0×10^9/l, Platelets 400×10^9/l, ESR 35 mm in the first hour.

Biochemistry
Sodium 140 mmol/l, Potassium 3.3 mmol/l, Urea 5.0 mmol/l, Creatinine 90 µmol/l, Bilirubin 6.0 µmol/l, Aspartate aminotransferase 15 iu/l, Alkaline phosphatase 60 iu/l, Total protein 76 g/l, Albumin 41 g/l, Calcium 2.5 mmol/l, Phosphate 1.23 mmol/l, Creatinine kinase 35 iu/l, Glucose 6.0 mmol/l.

Other investigations:

T4 80 nmol/l, ANA and rheumatoid factor negative. Syphilis serology negative.
Urine dipstick — negative protein. No Bence–Jones proteins.
Lumbar puncture: CSF Glu 4.0 mmol/l, Protein 1.0 g/l, WBC 20 mm³, no fungi or microorganisms seen.
Chest X-ray, calcification and pleural thickening in both lung apices. Abdominal X-ray normal
CT head scan — cortical and cerebellar atrophy, no focal lesions seen.

Abdominal ultrasound — minimal ascites, normal sized liver, kidneys and spleen with normal architecture; no lymphadenopathy; the right ovary contained several cysts containing some calcification; the left ovary was not seen.

a) What is the most likely diagnosis?

b) What investigation would you perform next?

66 A A 25-year-old woman presents with acute renal failure. Diffuse interstitial shadowing is noted on CXR and she has marked arterial hypoxaemia. Pulmonary function tests are as follows: FEV 75%, VC 67%, FEV/VC 114%, DLCO 173%, KCO 275%, VA 62%.

a) What is the abnormality and what pathological process is occurring?

b) Give two possible causes in this patient.

B A 53-year-old man complains of difficulty in breathing, worse in the morning and sometimes waking him at night. Lung function tests are shown below: FEV 57%, VC 93%, FEV/VC 63%, TLCO 116%, KCO 145%, VA 80%. Spirometry post-bronchodilator: FEV 92%, VC 101%, FEV/VC 72 (93%)

a) What is the diagnosis?

67 A 43-year-old woman presents with exertional shortness of breath. She swims regularly, and her symptoms are particularly marked when swimming breast stroke. She has no impairment of normal daily activities. She does not smoke or drink, and there is no previous medical history of note.

On examination she looks well, has a body mass index of 27 kg/m², and no cyanosis, oedema or clubbing. Pulse 70 bpm (regular); BP 115/80 mmHg; JVP normal; heart and lung examination normal. No abdominal masses or fluid are detected. Neurological examination is also normal.

A wide range of investigations are performed:

Urea and electrolytes, FBC, liver function tests normal.

Chest X-ray and CT of chest scan: normal, erect FEV and FVC and TLCO normal. Baseline oxygen saturation: 97%.

Resting and exercise ECGs: normal.

a) What is the likely diagnosis?

b) What further tests should be performed?

68 A 65-year-old man was seen in outpatients with a 3-month history of malaise, headache, myalgia, scalp tenderness, fever and weight loss. On examination vision was normal, both carotid arteries were tender to palpation. Routine blood investigations were normal but the ESR was elevated at 100 mm in the first hour. A clinical diagnosis of giant-cell arteritis was made and he was treated with 60 mg of prednisolone a day. Two months later he was still on 60 mg of prednisolone a day and his symptoms had not improved.

Investigations:

Hb	9.8 g/dl
MCV	82 fl
WBC	9×10^9/l
Platelets	260×10^9/l
ESR	123 mm in the first hour
Sodium	140 mmol/l
Potassium	4 mmol/l
Urea	3.7 mmol/l
Albumin	37 g/l
Bilirubin	23 µmol/l
Aspartate amino-transferase	26 iu/l
Urine dipstick	protein++, blood +++

a) Do you agree with the initial diagnosis?
b) What diagnosis would you consider?

69 A 44-year-old mother of three was referred from Greece for further treatment and investigation of possible systemic vasculitis. She presented 1 year previously with pain in her ankles and calves, particularly marked on exertion. She had a history of Raynaud's, had had two previous miscarriages, regular and heavy menstrual periods, and drank 2 bottles of Retsina per week. She was a life-long smoker.
On examination no pulses were felt below the femoral on the right, and the dorsalis pedis and posterior tibial were absent on the left. Blood pressure was normal and the peripheral perfusion was poor. She had localized ischaemia of the third toe on the right, with an interdigital infection.

Investigations:

Hb 10.4×10^9/l, MCV 74 fl, ESR 23 mm/h, and CRP 17 mg/l. Biochemical profile and blood glucose were normal. APTT and PT were normal.
No antibodies to double stranded DNA were detectable; ANA was positive with a titre of 1/40; complement levels normal.

a) What is the likely diagnosis?
b) What other investigations would you perform?
c) What other possibilities should be considered?

70 This patient has been admitted to the ITU with progressive deterioration after an influenza-like illness. Swan–Ganz and radial artery cannulae are in place.

	Sat O_2(%)	Press (mmHg)
SVC	48	
IVC	43	
mRA	47	Mean 22
RV	48	30/12
PA	47	33/16
PCWP		Mean 29
		V-wave 39
Radial artery	98	74/50

a) Why is the patient cyanosed?
b) Why is the superior vena cava blood so desaturated, and why is it less desaturated than the inferior vena cava blood?
c) What single measurement confers some grounds for hope of possible recovery?
d) Does the radial artery saturation surprise you? What is the explanation?

71 A 30-year-old woman was admitted with an upper gastrointestinal tract haemorrhage. She had had mild upper abdominal pain for 1 year; otherwise she was well. She was on no regular medication. She was unmarried, worked as a journalist, smoked 20 cigarettes per day and on average drank 2 glasses of wine per week.

On examination she was well tanned but had pale mucous membranes. There were two spider naevi on her upper trunk but no palmar erythema, jaundice or lymphadenopathy. Examination of the heart and lungs was normal. On palpation of her abdomen her liver was one finger-breadth below the costal margin and the tip of her spleen could be felt. Neurological examination was normal.

Investigations:

Hb	12.5 g/dl
WBC	5.5×10^9/l
Platelets	200×10^9/l
MCV	88 fl
ESR	40 mm in the first hour
Sodium	135 mmol/l
Potassium	4 mmol/l
Urea	5 mmol/l
Albumin	35 g/l
IgG	16 g/l
IgM	9 g/l
IgA	2 g/l
Calcium	1.9 mmol/l
Phosphate	0.6 mmol/l
Glucose	5.0 mmol/l

Bilirubin	12 µmol/l
Aspartate transaminase	30 iu/l
Alkaline phosphatase	300 iu/l
γ-GT	80 iu/l
Prothrombin time	12 s
Chest X-ray	normal
Abdominal X-ray	normal
Urinalysis	normal

a) Give the most likely underlying diagnosis.
b) What further investigations would you request?

72 An 87-year-old man presents with a 3-year history of intermittent diarrhoea. He denies abdominal pain and his appetite has been unimpaired but he has lost 2 stones in weight over this period. He has obstructive airways disease and a 30-year history of grand mal epilepsy which is well controlled by phenytoin. Seven years previously he underwent emergency surgery for acute abdominal pain and peritonitis. He lives alone and has a poor diet, including 2 pints of Guinness every day.

On examination he is pale and cachectic. Abdominal examination is normal apart from the presence of a central scar.

Investigations:

Hb	8.4 g/dl
WBC	4.3×10^9/l
Platelets	90×10^9/l
MCV	125 fl
Sodium	137 mmol/l
Potassium	4 mmol/l
Urea	4 mmol/l
Serum folate	22 µg/l
B_{12}	80 ng/l
Schilling test	5% pre-intrinsic factor
	6% post-intrinsic factor

a) What is the likely cause of the anaemia?
b) What further investigations would you perform to confirm this?

73 A 55-year-old man was referred with an 8-month history of tiredness and mild ankle oedema. Eight years ago he had had a small anterior myocardial infarction from which he had made an uneventful recovery; he had had prostatic cancer diagnosed 9 months ago and an anxiety state diagnosed 2 years before. His medication was fosfestrol 200 mg 8-hourly and atenolol 100 mg daily.

On examination his pulse was 55 regular, BP 120/60 mmHg, he had cold peripheries but was not cyanosed. There was no anaemia, jaundice or lymphadenopathy. The jugular venous pressure was visible on expiration. Palpation of the praecordium and first and second heart sounds were normal. He had mild ankle oedema and several inspiratory crackles at both lung bases. Examination of his neck, abdomen and nervous system were otherwise normal.

Investigations:

Hb	12 g/dl
WBC	$5.0 \times 10^9/l$
Sodium	139 mmol/l
Potassium	4 mmol/l
Urea	4.0 mmol/l
Creatinine	70 μmol/l
Albumin	35 g/l
T4	180 nmol/l
TSH	1.0 mU/l
Urinalysis	normal
CXR	normal heart size and clear lung fields
ECG	sinus rhythm, with normal QRS and T-wave inversion in leads V4–6.

a) What is the explanation for this patient's clinical problems?
b) What two investigations would you request?

74 A 52-year-old woman is admitted to casualty feeling unwell. She has a severe headache, which came on suddenly while she was watching television, and has vomited once. She is apyrexial, but has some neck stiffness and is rather drowsy. Pulse 100 sinus rhythm, BP 150/95 mmHg. She has no other focal neurological signs, and fundoscopy was normal.

a) What are the two main differential diagnoses? Which is the more likely, and why?
b) What is the most important initial investigation that is required? How will the results help to distinguish between the two main differential diagnoses?
c) What other tests should be performed urgently?
d) What is the commonest cause of this problem?
e) How would you manage this patient?

75 A 36-year-old housewife was admitted with 3-month history of difficulty in walking. She complained that her legs felt stiff and weak but she was otherwise well and had no significant past medical history. Her periods had been irregular and heavy since the birth of her 18-month-old son. She smoked 20 cigarettes a day and drank 2 pints of stout a night.

On examination she avoided eye contact but higher mental function was normal. Gait was spastic in nature, tone was symmetrically increased in both legs, power was decreased in a pyramidal fashion, reflexes were brisk with bilateral clonus and extensor plantars. No sensory abnormality could be detected, abdominal reflexes were absent. Neurological examination of the arms and cranial nerves was normal. General examination was unremarkable.

Investigations:

Hb	8.3 g/dl
MCV	72 fl
MCH	26 pg
MCHC	28 g/dl
WBC	5×10^9/l
Platelets	237×10^9/l
ESR	5 mm in the first hour
Sodium	138 mmol/l
Potassium	4 mmol/l
Urea	4 mmol/l
Albumin	40 g/l
Calcium	2.7 mmol/l
Aspartate amino-transferase	23 iu/l
Alkaline phosphatase	123 iu/l
Bilirubin	8 μmol/l
Chest X-ray	well-defined circular lesion overlying the left pulmonary artery
Thoracic spine X-ray	normal
Lung function tests	low DLCO and KCO (for Hb 8.3 g/dl)

a) Give a differential diagnosis. What is the most likely diagnosis?
b) What is the single most important investigation to perform? List three other investigations you would perform.

76 A A 65-year-old woman develops persistent diarrhoea. On examination she appears to have a migratory erythematous rash over her legs.

Investigations:

Hb	9 g/dl
WBC	$11 \times 10^9/l$
Platelets	$230 \times 10^9/l$
Glucose	10 mmol/l

a) Give a unifying diagnosis.
b) How would you confirm your diagnosis?
c) How would you manage the patient?

B A 35-year-old male solicitor is referred by his GP. He was diagnosed as being hypertensive 1 year ago and despite drug treatment including β-blockers, calcium antagonists and an ACE inhibitor, his blood pressure remains elevated. He drinks 4 pints of beer per day and smokes 2 cigars every evening.

In the clinic, supine blood pressure is recorded as 210/110 mmHg. Fundi — grade III retinopathy. The rest of the examination is normal.

Investigations:

Sodium	148 mmol/l
Potassium	3.0 mmol/l
Bicarbonate	32 mmol/l
Urea	4 mmol/l
Glucose	4 mmol/l
Urine	negative protein

a) What is the likely diagnosis?
b) What further investigations are indicated?

77 The affected members in this family were below the 3rd centile in height and had a plasma phosphate consistently below 0.45 mmol/l; their alkaline phosphatase was between 150 and 200 iu/l and their calcium was within the normal range.

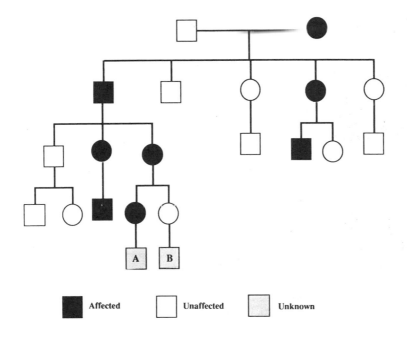

Affected   Unaffected   Unknown

a) What is the diagnosis? How is the defect inherited?
b) What is the risk of A and B being affected?

78 A 26-year-old woman presents to casualty after a series of grand mal fits. She had been well until the onset of fits 12 hours previously. On examination she has a temperature of 38°C, pulse 90, blood pressure 135/90 mmHg. Neurologically she is alert with a left VI nerve palsy and upper motor weakness of the right arm.

Investigations:

Hb	9.7 g/dl
WBC	8.9×10^9/l
Platelets	20×10^9/l
Blood film	red cell fragmentation
PT	16 s
APTT	47 s
Fibrinogen	1.5 g/l
TT	36 s
FDPs	1:1240
Sodium	134 mmol/l
Potassium	5.2 mmol/l
Urea	26 mmol/l
Creatinine	364 μmol/l
Urine microscopy	blood++, protein++

a) What is the likely diagnosis?

79

	Sat O$_2$(%)	Press (mmHg)
mRA		Mean 14
PA		27/12
PACW		Mean 24
Femoral artery	96	

This patient has a pansystolic murmur which developed 3 days after a myocardial infarction. There is a Swan–Ganz catheter in place. A femoral blood sample shows arterial saturation.

a) Can the patient lie flat?
b) What two diagnoses must be differentiated?
c) What simple measurement can be made without further cannulation to distinguish between these?
d) What effect will inspiration have on the murmur?

80 A 50-year-old man was unable to work because of lethargy and depression. He was hypertensive and had mild angina. One year before he had been involved in a road traffic accident and sustained a head injury. He was pursuing an insurance claim and attributed his symptoms to anxiety. His medication was methyldopa 250 mg 12-hourly, Moduretic two tablets daily and GTN when required.

On examination he was pale, had thinning of his frontal hair and eyebrows and had lost most of his axillary and pubic hair. His neck, heart and lungs were normal. BP lying 120/70 mmHg, standing 105/60 mmHg. Neurological examination was normal apart from slow relaxation of his ankle jerks.

Investigations:

Hb	13 g/dl
WBC	$9 \times 10^9/l$
ESR	10 mm in the first hour
Sodium	126 mmol/l
Potassium	3.8 mmol/l
Urea	6 mmol/l
Albumin	40 g/l
Aspartate amino-transferase	30 iu/l
Alkaline phosphatase	100 iu/l
Bilirubin	5.5 μmol/l
Chest X-ray	normal
ECG	small voltage complexes
T4	50 nmol/l, TSH 1.0 mU/l
Anti-microsomal antibodies	+1/1250

a) What is the diagnosis?
b) What investigations would you suggest?
c) What treatment and advice would you give him about his condition?

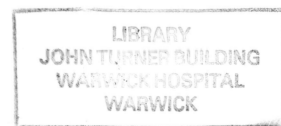

81 A 15-year-old girl presents with a 2-month history of fatigue. She commenced her periods 18 months previously and these have recently become heavy. On three occasions in the past her mother has commented that she 'looks yellow'. Her father, who no longer lives at home, was diagnosed in his youth as having recurrent anaemia. She has no siblings and is on no medication. On examination she is pale, and abdominal examination reveals 2 cm splenomegaly.

Investigations:

Hb	6.6 g/dl
WBC	8.4×10^9/l
Platelets	385×10^9/l
Reticulocytosis	10%
Direct Coombs' test	negative
Sodium	141 mmol/l
Potassium	4.9 mmol/l
Urea	4.3 mmol/l
Bilirubin	38 μmol/l
Aspartate transaminase	69 iu/l
Alkaline phosphatase	119 iu/l
Haptoglobins	not detected
Urinary haemosiderin	absent

a) What is the likely diagnosis and how would you investigate further?

82 A 38-year-old woman presents with a 2-day history of a painful, swollen right leg. Eight years previously she had had a similar episode which spontaneously resolved. Three weeks previously she had had an upper respiratory tract infection for which she was prescribed amoxycillin by her family doctor. Over the previous 3 years she had noticed the occasional passing of dark urine, particularly first thing in the morning. This, coupled with a complaint of intermittent colicky abdominal pain, led her family doctor to perform an IVU and abdominal ultrasound 1 year ago, both of which were normal. Her father died at the age of 50 from a cerebrovascular accident and there is a strong family history of hypertension. She smokes 20 cigarettes a day, drinks no alcohol and is on no regular medication.

On examination she is pyrexial 38.2°C, normotensive and has a tense, erythematous, painful, swollen left calf.

Investigations:

Hb	8.9 g/dl
WBC	2.3 × 10⁹/l (40% neutrophils)
Platelets	43 × 10⁹/l
Sodium	143 mmol/l
Potassium	3.6 mmol/l
Urea	4.3 mmol/l
Bilirubin	12 µmol/l
Aspartate amino-transferase	32 iu/l
Alkaline phosphatase	124 iu/l
PT	12 s
APTT	37 s
Fibrinogen	2.6 g/l
Thrombin time	15 s

a) What is the likely diagnosis?
b) How would you confirm your diagnosis?

83 A 64-year-old Somali woman has a 6-month history of 2-stone weight loss and episodic severe colickly abdominal pain, not associated with meals, posture or bowel habit.

Investigations:

Sodium	125 mmol/l
Potassium	6.4 mmol/l
Urea	14 mmol/l
Calcium	2.76 mmol/l
Glucose	3.3 mmol/l
T4	34 nmol/l
TSH	24 mU/l
Thyroid microsomal antibodies	not detected

a) What is the diagnosis?
b) What treatment is indicated for the endocrine abnormalities?

84 This is the report of an exercise tolerance test. Standard Bruce protocol was used. The test was terminated at 5 minutes 22 seconds with chest pain.

a) What is the most likely pathology underlying this change?
b) The patient's resting blood pressure on no treatment is 110/70. What other condition must be considered?
c) What two important investigations should be considered?

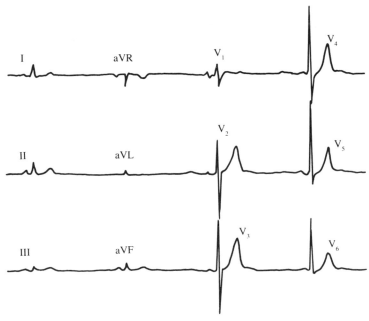

Pre-exercise ECG   0.75 cm = 1 mV

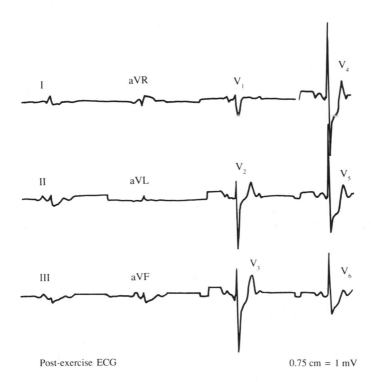

I   aVR V_1 V_4

II   aVL V_2 V_5

III   aVF V_3 V_6

Post-exercise ECG   0.75 cm = 1 mV

85 A 28-year-old man with a 6-year history of Crohn's disease has a 6-month history of frequent offensive loose stools and weight loss of 9 kg. General examination is unremarkable and sigmoidoscopy shows normal mucosa to the rectosigmoid junction, with views partially obscured by loose faeces and mucus.

Investigations:

Sodium	136 mmol/l
Potassium	4.2 mmol/l
Urea	4.4 mmol/l
Creatinine	110 μmol/l
Calcium	2.18 mmol/l
Albumin	34 g/l
Hb	13.2 g/dl
MCV	106 fl
PTT	22 s
3 day faecal fat	22 mmol/24 hours
Vit B_{12}	64 ng/l

Schilling test:

24-hr urine radioactivity minus IF: low
24-hr urine radioactivity plus IF: low
24-hr urine vol 1220 ml
24-hr urine creatinine 7.8 g/l

$^{14}CO_2$ breath test	^{14}C in breath — high
	^{14}C in faeces — low

a) What is the likely explanation for the results of the Schilling test?

86 A A 36-year-old Indian man has the following blood count on a routine check-up:

Hb	12.8 g/dl
MCV	64 fl
MCH	24 pg
MCHC	26 g/dl
WBC	5.6×10^9/l
Platelets	237×10^9/l
Hb electrophoresis	A A2 F

a) What is the cause of the haematological abnormalities?
b) What action would you take?

B The following results are obtained in a 32-year-old woman with galactorrhoea:

Sodium	136 mmol/l
Potassium	5.5 mmol/l
Bicarbonate	18 mmol/l
Calcium (corrected)	2.04 mmol/l
Hb	8.6 g/dl
MCV	92 fl
MCH	32 pg
T4	48 nmol/l
TSH	2.4 mU/l

a) What is this woman's primary condition?

Question 87

87 **A** A 36-year-old man presents with a sudden history of lower abdominal pain and weakness of the right leg. Eight years previously he had had an aortic valve replacement. Since then he has been maintained on warfarin and propranolol until 2 weeks prior to presentation when the propranolol had been changed to a different antiarrhythmic agent. On examination he is in pain. In the cardiovascular system he has an ejection systolic murmur maximal at the left sternal edge.

Neurologically he has a flaccid right leg with loss of sensation to pinprick and light touch over the lateral aspect of the right thigh. The right patellar reflex is absent.

Investigations:

Hb	9.6 g/dl
WBC	7.4×10^9/l
Platelets	374×10^9/l
Sodium	145 mmol/l
Potassium	4 mmol/l
Urea	4.7 mmol/l
Bilirubin	23 µmol/l
Aspartate amino-transferase	25 iu/l
Alkaline phosphatase	123 iu/l
PT	93 s
APTT	48 s
Fibrinogen	3.1 g/l

a) What is the likely diagnosis and how would you treat this man?

B A 43-year-old woman presents with a history of increasing tiredness. Seven years previously she was successfully treated with combined chemotherapy and radiotherapy for stage IV Hodgkin's disease.

Investigations:

Hb	10.2 g/dl
WBC	3.4×10^9/l, neutrophils 34%, Pelger cells and occasional blasts
Platelets	49×10^9/l
MCV	108 fl

a) What is the likely cause of her anaemia?

88 This is the ECG of a 14-year-old boy who has recurrent dizzy spells.

a) What is the diagnosis?

b) What two arrhythmias may underlie the dizzy spells? What is the danger of the less common of the two?

c) Give three other causes of a positive R-wave in lead V1.

Limb leads

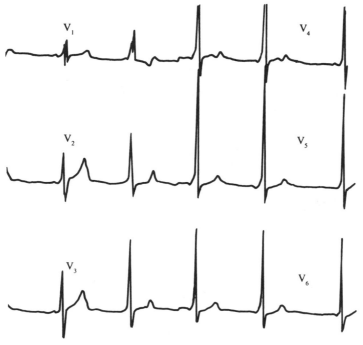

Chest leads

89 A A 75-year-old man presents with tiredness. On examination he is pale, has widespread lymphadenopathy and a 6 cm spleen.

Investigations:

Hb	7.6 g/dl
WBC	28 × 10⁹/l — 92% lymphocytes
Platelets	52 × 10⁹/l
Blood film	polychromasia and spherocytes
Reticulocytes	8%
Serum haptoglobins	undetected

a) What is the likely diagnosis?
b) How would you confirm your diagnosis?

B Investigations from a 5-year-old child:

PT	14 s
APPT	80 s
TT	12 s
Fibrinogen	3.5 g
Bleeding time	7 minutes

a) What is the likely diagnosis?
b) What are the likely complications?

90 A 59-year-old woman presents to outpatients with increasing tiredness and thirst. She has frequent epigastric pain and has woken on three occasions in the night with such pain in the last week.

Investigations:

Hb	11.3 g/dl
WBC	6.4 × 10⁹/l
Platelets	264 × 10⁹/l
ESR	9 mm in the first hour
Sodium	136 mmol/l
Potassium	4.3 mmol/l
Urea	11.5 mmol/l
Creatinine	140 μmol/l
Calcium	3.25 mmol/l
Phosphate	0.72 mmol/l
Chloride	117 mmol/l
Bicarbonate	12 mmol/l
Alkaline phosphatase	170 iu/l
Albumin	40 g/l

a) What is the likely diagnosis? What is the significance of the epigastric pain?
b) How do these patients usually present?
c) How would you confirm your diagnosis?
d) Give a differential diagnosis.

91 A 40-year-old woman presents with a 3-month history of polyarthralgia and progressive difficulty climbing stairs.

Investigations:

Hb	13 g/dl
WBC	5×10^9/l
Platelets	250×10^9/l
ESR	36 mm in the first hour
Urea	5 mmol/l
Creatinine	130 mmol/l
Albumin	40 g/l
Aspartate amino-transferase	65 iu/l
Bilirubin	14 µmol/l
Alkaline phosphatase	120 iu/l
IgG	28 g/l
T4	80 nmol/l
Closed muscle biopsy	Normal

EMG Spontaneous fibrillation, high-frequency repetitive discharges and polyphasic short small motor-unit potentials

a) What is the most likely diagnosis?

92 a) Why was this glucose tolerance test performed on this 60-year-old man?

b) What conclusions may be drawn from it?

Time *min*	Blood glucose *mmol/l*	Growth hormone *ng/l*
0	8	12
30	13	13
60	16	11
90	12	12
120	10	12.5

Growth hormone normal basal value <3ng/ml.

93 A A 62-year-old man has been treated with twice weekly haemodialysis for chronic renal failure secondary to reflux nephropathy. A subtotal parathyroidectomy had successfully been performed 3 years earlier.

He complains of aching lower back pain and his wife reminds him that he has become increasingly forgetful of late. Medication includes iron and folic acid supplements, aluminium hydroxide and nifedipine.

Investigations:

Sodium	140 mmol/l
Potassium	4.5 mmol/l
Urea	24 mmol/l
Creatinine	560 µmol/l
Calcium	2.4 mmol/l
Phosphate	1.4 mmol/l
Alkaline phosphatase	120 iu/l
PTH	undetectable
Radiological survey	mild demineralization only

a) What is the likely diagnosis?
b) What treatment would you recommend?

B A 10-year-old boy is admitted for investigation. His mother has noted that he has become progressively clumsy. On examination he is alert and orientated. Abnormal findings were a right-sided intention tremor and right-sided nystagmus.

Investigations:

Hb	16 g/dl
WBC	6×10^9/l
Platelets	225×10^9/l
PCV	55%
Urea and electrolytes	normal

a) The history and signs point to a diagnosis in which part of the brain?
b) Give one unifying diagnosis.

94 A 75-year-old man is found lying on the floor of his house. On admission he is hypothermic, bradycardic, and peripherally shut down. Electrocardiogram shows sinus bradycardia with ST elevation in leads II, III and AVF. Emergency electrolytes show:

Sodium	135 mmol/l
Potassium	5.0 mmol/l
Bicarbonate	12 mmol/l
Chloride	100 mmol/l
Urea	7.5 mmol/l

a) Comment on the biochemistry and how you would confirm your diagnosis.

95 This is the M-mode echocardiogram of a 40-year-old woman.
   a) What disease causes this valve lesion?
   b) What is structure A?
   c) Describe two abnormalities of structure B.
   d) What physical sign would coincide with line C?

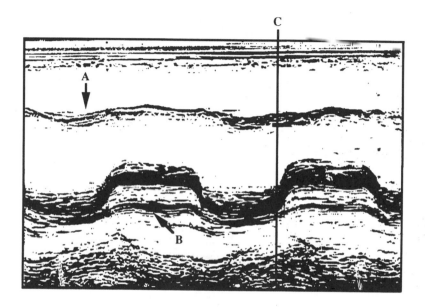

96 A 60-year-old man was admitted with a 4-day history of fever, myalgia and headache. Two days before admission the patient had developed abdominal pain and had 3 loose stools. The GP was called by his wife when he became disorientated and confused. He had had no serious illnesses in the past and took no regular medication. He was a non-smoker and drank approximately one pint of beer a day.

Examination: Temperature 40°C; pulse 100 regular, BP 120/70 mmHg, respiration rate 24/min. The patient was clinically disorientated but specific examination of the nervous system was normal apart from mild neck stiffness. There was no anaemia, cyanosis, rash, lymphadenopathy or jaundice. Crackles were heard at his right base and in the left mid-zone. Examination of the heart was normal. There was diffuse abdominal tenderness and his liver edge could be felt two finger-breadths below the costal margin in the mid-clavicular line.

Investigations:

Hb	13.5 g/dl
WBC	15×10^9/l — neutrophils 95%, lymphocytes 4%
Platelets	300×10^9/l
ESR	110 mm in the first hour
Sodium	127 mmol/l
Potassium	3.8 mmol/l
Urea	10.0 mmol/l
Creatinine	110 µmol/l
Albumin	38 g/l
Calcium	1.9 mmol/l
Phosphate	0.8 mmol/l
Bilirubin	14 µmol/l
Aspartate transaminase	80 iu/l
Alkaline phosphatase	200 iu/l
Glucose	5.0 mmol/l
pH	7.4
pO_2	9.0 kPa
pCO_2	4.0 kPa
Chest X-ray	increased shadowing in the right base and a small pleural effusion
CSF	Glucose 4.0 mmol/l, protein 0.8 g/l, <3 WBC/mm³ No bacteria seen

Routine cultures of blood, urine and CSF, and throat washings and stool were negative. The patient was started on intravenous amoxycillin but continued to deteriorate.

a) What is the most likely diagnosis?
b) How would you confirm your diagnosis?
c) How would you treat this patient?

97 A 60-year-old woman presented with abdominal pain. She had been unwell for 2–3 weeks and felt 'weak'. For 3 weeks she had had intermittent sharp pains in her left upper quadrant and more recently a dull ache in her left iliac fossa. A week before admission she developed night sweats. There had been several episodes when she had become dizzy and confused and on one occasion she had lost vision in her left eye. She had a number of vague rheumatic symptoms but no early morning stiffness, headaches or jaw claudication. In the past she had had a hysterectomy and a cholecystectomy. She took no regular medication. There was no family history of significant disease.

Temperature 39°C, pulse 120, BP 140/60 mmHg, respiratory rate 40/min. She had no rash, lymphadenopathy or clubbing. Two small conjunctival haemorrhages were visible. Examination of her respiratory system was unremarkable. Her heart sounds were normal; a soft pansystolic murmur could be heard only at the apex. There was a tender pulsatile mass in the left iliac fossa and the spleen was palpable and tender. Neurological examination was normal. The peripheral pulses were present and equal. There were no bruits.

Investigations:

Hb	11 g/dl
WBC	8.0×10^9/l
Platelets	300×10^9/l
ESR	50 mm in the first hour
Sodium	140 mmol/l
Potassium	4.0 mmol/l
Urea	9 mmol/l
Creatinine	90 μmol/l
Albumin	30 g/l
Bilirubin	8.0 μmol/l
Aspartate amino-transferase	40 iu/l
Alkaline phosphatase	140 iu/l
Calcium	2.0 mmol/l
Chest X-ray and abdominal X-rays	normal
ECG	sinus tachycardia
Urinalysis	protein +; blood +, no casts seen

An ultrasound of the abdomen showed a large spleen with wedge-shaped areas of increased density.

a) What is the most likely diagnosis?
b) Suggest three investigations.

98 An anxious 20-year-old woman presented with mild shortness of breath on exertion, which had come on gradually over several months. The symptoms were intermittent but seemed to be worse in the evening. Her husband complained that during the episodes she appeared depressed and her speech was slurred. She had been treated for depression in the past and recently had been started on lorazepam by her GP for anxiety.

On examination in outpatients she looked very well. There was no anaemia, cyanosis, clubbing, jaundice or oedema. Examination of her respiratory and cardiovascular system was normal. Abdominal examination was normal. The cranial nerves, muscle tone, power, coordination and tendon reflexes were normal. Sensation was intact.

Investigations:

FBC	normal
ESR	20 mm in the first hour
Electrolytes and liver function tests	normal
Chest X-ray	normal
Lung function tests	normal

a) What is the most likely diagnosis?
b) What tests would you perform?

99 Part 1 This is the M-mode echocardiograph at the level of mid left ventricle. Centimetre marks are shown.

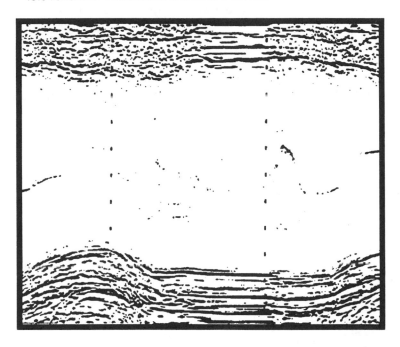

Part 2 This is the apical doppler signal across the aortic valve.

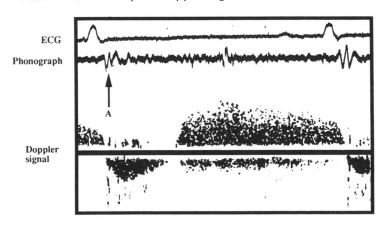

a) What abnormality is demonstrated in the left ventricle?
b) What is A on the phonocardiogram?
c) During which phase of the cardiac cycle is the dominant doppler signal shown and is it towards or away from the apex?
d) What is the cause of the left ventricular abnormality?

100 A 63-year-old man who lived alone was referred with a short history of confusion and urinary incontinence. He had mild maturity-onset diabetes controlled by diet alone and was hypertensive. Regular treatment included bendrofluazide and propranolol 40 mg 12-hourly. Eighteen months ago he had had meningococcal meningitis which had responded well to penicillin. He had no history of head injury and no history of epilepsy. He was a lifelong non-smoker and did not drink alcohol. Although he lived alone he had good support from his daughter who lived in the same street and provided his meals.

Temperature was 37°C, pulse 70 regular, BP 140/70 mmHg. On examination he was alert and orientated in person but not in time or location. He was unable to remember simple sentences, and confabulated. His memory of recent events was poor. He was unable to perform simple arithmetic. There was no evidence of dysphasia, apraxia, or agnosia. There was no neck stiffness and no papilloedema. The cranial nerves were normal; examination of limbs revealed no motor or sensory signs. Coordination in his lower limbs was poor; he had a wide-based, fixed-footed gait and tended to fall unless he had assistance.

Examination of his chest and abdomen was unremarkable.

Investigations:

Urinalysis	normal
Sodium	137 mmol/l
Potassium	3.7 mmol/l
Urea	7 mmol/l
Calcium	2.3 mmol/l
Albumin	38 g/l
Total protein	75 g/l
Urate	6.0 mmol/l
WBC	7×10^9/l
Platelets	400×10^9/l
ESR	30 mm in the first hour
B_{12} and folate	normal
CRP	8 mg/l
VDRL	neg
T4	90 nmol/l
TSH	2.0 mU/l
CXR and skull X-ray	normal

a) What is the most likely diagnosis?
b) What is the treatment and what complications may follow?

101 A young man is admitted because he is breathless.

PEFR	200 l/min
Blood gases	air
pH	7.5
pO_2	9 kPa
pCO_2	3.5 kPa
Bicarbonate	12 mmol/l

a) What are the abnormalities and how would you correct them?

Later his blood gases on 40% oxygen are:

pH	7.28
pO_2	8 kPa
pCO_2	6.5
Bicarbonate	17 mmol/l

b) What has happened? Give a differential diagnosis. What treatment would you consider?

102 This is an M-mode echocardiogram through the aortic root (space A).
   a) What is B?
   b) What is causing B?
   c) What is C and is it normal?
   d) The underlying disease is rheumatic heart disease — what can be deduced about the mitral valve?

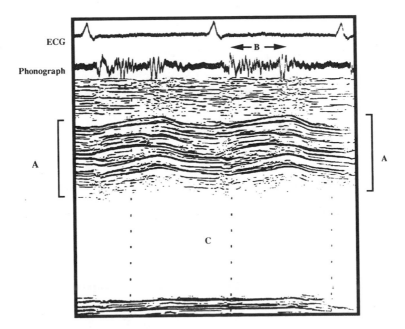

103 A 12-year-old boy developed recurrent upper abdominal pain
and intermittent diarrhoea after returning from a short holiday
with his school to Leningrad. The stools were bulky, pale and
offensive. He had no fever and had an excellent appetite. In the
past he had had whooping cough and since then had regular
attacks of bronchitis during the winter, but was able to play
games and had little time off school.

On examination he had no rash, anaemia, clubbing,
lymphadenopathy or jaundice. His height was on the 50th centile
and weight 60% of that predicted for an average boy of his age.
His two other siblings were both within the normal range.
Examination of the cardiovascular system was normal.
Examination of the chest revealed crackles at his left base and
right mid-zone. On palpation his abdomen was soft and there
was no organomegaly. His right colon was easily palpable and
loaded with faeces. Examination of the CNS was normal.

Investigations:

Hb	13 g/dl
WBC	$9 \times 10^9/l$
Platelets	$400 \times 10^9/l$
ESR	50 mm in the first hour
Sodium	137 mmol/l
Potassium	4.1 mmol/l
Urea	6 mmol/l
Albumin	25 g/l
Total protein	70 g/l
B_{12}	300 ng/l
Folate	2 µg/l
Iron	17 µmol/l
TIBC	50 µmol/l
Faecal fat excretion	28 mmol/l

CXR small patches of atelectasis in the left base. AXR a dilated
colon loaded with faeces.

a) What is the most likely diagnosis?
b) What investigations would you request?

104 A 65-year-old man was reviewed in clinic. He complained of increased shortness of breath on exertion and was breathless walking up two flights of stairs. Recently he had felt increasingly tired, with myalgia and pain in a number of his joints but no swelling or stiffness. His GP had increased his dose of frusemide without apparent benefit. Seven years previously he had had aortic valve replacement for aortic regurgitation. A second Starr–Edwards prosthesis was inserted 3 years after an episode of infective endocarditis. Two years later he had developed atrial fibrillation which was controlled by digoxin and verapamil; on examination, crepitations were heard in his lung bases and 40 mg of frusemide was started. A right heart catheter was passed and a normal wedge pressure recorded. An echocardiogram indicated that the aortic prosthesis was functioning well and the other heart valves were normal. The atrial fibrillation had become difficult to control with digoxin and verapamil 6 months ago and they had been replaced with amiodarone, with marked symptomatic improvement. He was a lifelong non-smoker and had no exposure to occupational dusts or fumes.

Now on examination he was warm but peripherally cyanosed. Pulse 80 irregularly irregular, blood pressure 110/70, JVP visible. The cardiac apex beat was not palpable and there were no abnormal heaves or thrills. Auscultation revealed prosthetic heart sounds only. There were fine inspiratory crackles audible in the lower zones of both lungs.

A chest X-ray showed diffuse linear shadowing in both lower zones. The ECG had not changed from previous visits and showed atrial fibrillation with left bundle branch block.

Investigations:

Hb	15 g/l
WBC	8×10^9/l
Platelets	300×10^9/l
ESR	80 mm in the first hour
Sodium	135 mmol/l
Potassium	3.5 mmol/l
Urea	12 mmol/l
Creatinine	90 μmol/l
Albumin	45 g/l
Total protein	90 g/l
Aspartate transaminase	40 iu/l
Alkaline phosphatase	120 iu/l
Bilirubin	10 μmol/l
Rheumatoid factor	1/80
ANA positive	1/40
PEFR	450
FEV1	90%
FVC	70%

a) What is the most likely cause of the breathlessness?
b) What three investigations would you arrange?

105 This patient has recurrent syncope.
   a) Identify three abnormalities.
   b) How is the ventricular mass depolarised?
   c) What underlies the syncope and what treatment is indicated?

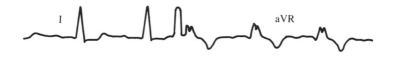

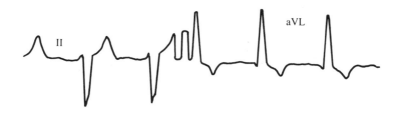

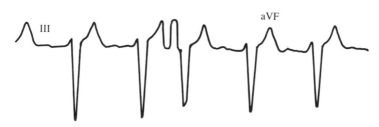

Limb leads

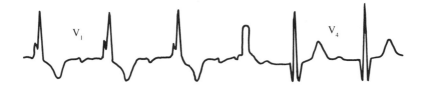

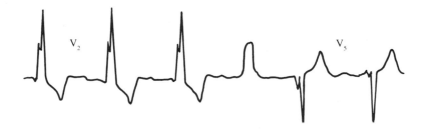

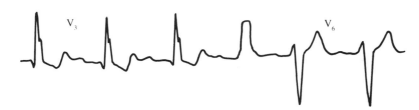

Chest leads

20 mm/sec; 0.8 cm/mV

106 A woman aged 27 years, in the 30th week of her first pregnancy, complained of tiredness and breathlessness on exertion. She had had no chest pain, cough or haemoptysis but had had mild facial flushing. She had no history of foreign travel and was not exposed to hazardous fumes in the factory where she worked. There was no family history of illness. She had not had any serious illnesses in the past. She was a non-smoker who drank little alcohol and had never abused drugs. She had taken the oral contraceptive pill for 8 years before deciding to become pregnant.

On examination, she looked pale; her hands and feet were cold and cyanosed. She was not anaemic or clubbed. Pulse of 90, blood pressure 90/65 mmHg with no elevation of the jugular venous pressure. She had a palpable right ventricular heave. On auscultation a loud pulmonary second sound and a soft fourth heart sound could be heard. Her lung fields were clear. There was mild pitting oedema in both ankles.

Investigations:

Hb	14 g/dl
WBC	5.6×10^9/l
Platelets	400×10^9/l
Sodium	139 mmol/l
Potassium	3.9 mmol/l
Urea	5.9 mmol/l
Albumin	45 g/l
Total protein	75 g/l
Aspartate transaminase	36 iu/l
Alkaline phosphatase	120 iu/l
Bilirubin	4.5 µmol/l
ESR	30 mm in the first hour
CRP	10 mg/l
T4	80 nmol/l
TSH	2.0 mU/l

FEV_1 90%, FVC 100%, TLCO 95%, VA 90%, KCO 95%; CXR prominent pulmonary arteries, lung fields clear.

a) Give the two differential diagnoses.
b) What four investigations would you request?

Question 107

107A A 48-year-old woman was referred to casualty with headaches and somnolence. The headaches were diffuse and were worse on waking. The symptoms had begun 5 days earlier following an influenza-like illness. She had had mild breathlessness on exertion for several years which she attributed to her increasing weight and smoking 20 cigarettes per day. She had no serious medical problems in the past and took no regular medication.

On examination she was alert, had no anaemia or cyanosis. Her weight was 125 kg. Examination of her cardiorespiratory system was normal. Examination of her central nervous system was normal. There was no neck stiffness and her fundi were clear.

Investigations:

CXR	normal
Blood gases	air
pH	7.4
pO_2	10.5 kPa
pCO_2	6.5 kPa
Bicarbonate	32 mmol/l

a) What is the diagnosis?
b) What treatment would you suggest?

B A 26-year-old woman attends her GP with cystitis, for which he prescribes an empirical course of trimethoprim. Five days later her symptoms persist and she complains of nausea and occasional vomiting. In addition to sending an MSU for culture, the GP checks her serum biochemistry, the results of which are:

Sodium	138 mmol/l
Potassium	4.4 mmol/l
Bicarbonate	21 mmol/l
Urea	5.6 mmol/l
Creatinine	183 µmol/l

a) What is the likely explanation for the patient's biochemical abnormality?

108 A 41-year-old man had received a renal transplant 3 years previously. He was taking prednisolone and cyclosporin, and his graft was functioning normally. He presents to the clinic with a 2-month history of intermittent headache, nausea, dizziness, difficulty concentrating at work, and numbness over the left side of his face.

On examination — pulse 80; BP 130/70; T 38°C; mild neck stiffness; reduced sensation over the lower part of his face on the left; generalized hyperreflexia and upgoing plantar reflexes on both sides.

Investigations:

FBC normal, ESR 11 mm/hour.

MRI scan of the brain demonstrated no abnormality.

Lumbar puncture: CSF pressure 26 cm, protein 1.2 g.

WBC 190 cells/mm³ — 80% lymphocytes. Glucose 1.5 mmol/l (plasma glucose 5.6 mmol/l).

No organisms seen on routine Gram stain of the CSF.

a) Suggest two likely diagnoses.
b) What further tests should be performed on the CSF?
c) What treatment would you recommend?

109A A 55-year-old woman was found during the course of a routine medical examination to have a monoclonal band on protein electrophoresis.

Investigations:

IgG	20 g/l
IgM	0.8 g/l
IgA	2.5 g/l
Albumin	38 g/l
Calcium	2.4 mmol/l
Alkaline phosphatase	125 iu/l
Hb	12.9 g/dl
WBC	$5.7 \times 10^9/l$
Platelets	$267 \times 10^9/l$
ESR	45 mm in the first hour
Bence–Jones protein	negative
Bone marrow	3% plasma cells
Skeletal survey	normal

a) What diagnosis would you attach to her?
b) How would you manage her?

B A 45-year-old smoker complains of tiredness and weakness.

Investigations:

Blood pressure	180/110 mmHg
Sodium	140 mmol/l
Potassium	2.8 mmol/l
Bicarbonate	32 mmol/l
Urea	5 mmol/l
Glucose	12 mmol/l

a) What is the probable diagnosis?
b) What two investigations would you perform to confirm your diagnosis?

110 A 70-year-old man is admitted with exertional dyspnoea and bilateral leg oedema. He gives a 3-month history of bilateral numbness and tingling of the fingers.

Investigations:

Hb	11.8 g/dl
WBC	$5 \times 10^9/l$
Platelets	$350 \times 10^9/l$
ESR	98 mm in the first hour
Urea	8 mmol/l
Creatinine	130 μmol/l
Uric acid	0.5 mmol/l
Albumin	20 g/l
Alkaline phosphatase	100 iu/l
Aspartate amino-transferase	25 iu/l
Plasma electrophoresis	IgG monoclonal protein with immune paresis
24-hour protein excretion	8 g
ECG	low voltage complexes with 2:1 heart block

a) What is the likely underlying diagnosis?
b) Why is the patient short of breath and oedematous?

111 A 66-year-old man has attended his GP with a 3-year history of late-onset asthma and more recent exertional angina and intermittent claudication. He attends the surgery with a 3-week history of mild dyspnoea on exertion. Examination confirms a moderate expiratory wheeze, and a peak flow reading of 230 l/min is obtained. The GP prescribes a 1-week course of ampicillin in addition to his usual Ventolin inhaler. One week later the patient returns with no improvement. On examination, his temperature is 37.4°C. He has widespread expiratory wheezes. His blood pressure is 155/102. He has a number of purpuric lesions on his feet.

Investigations:

Hb	12 g/dl
WBC	11.8×10^9/l
Neutrophils	7.2×10^9/l
Lymphocytes	1.4×10^9/l
Eosinophils	3×10^9/l
Urea	13.6 mmol/l
Creatinine	210 µmol/l
FEV1	2.8 l
FVC	4.9 l
Urinalysis	Protein++
	blood — non-haemolysed trace
Urine microscopy	20 white cells/hpf
	scanty granular casts.

a) What is the probable diagnosis?
b) What clinical features are suggestive of this diagnosis?
c) Give two other causes of renal impairment associated with eosinophilia.

112 A The following results are obtained in a 72-year-old smoker.

Sodium	119 mmol/l
Potassium	3.6 mmol/l
Blood uric acid	0.08 mmol/l
Urea	4.5 mmol/l
Glucose	5.2 mmol/l
Urinary sodium	54 mmol/l
Urinary osmolality	456 mosm/kg

a) What pathology is suggested by these results?
b) What are the three principles of treatment?

B What investigation is indicated to explain this patient's hyponatraemia?

Sodium	118 mmol/l
Potassium	4.3 mmol/l
Urea	4.8 mmol/l
Glucose	4.6 mmol/l
Plasma osmolality	284 mOsmol/kg
Albumin	24 g/l
24-hour urinary protein	7.8 g

113 a) This patient has had a pacemaker inserted for two separate rhythm disturbances. What are they?

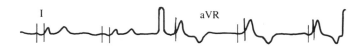

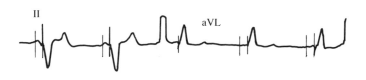

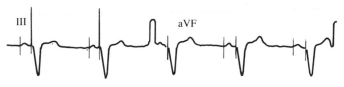

Limb leads

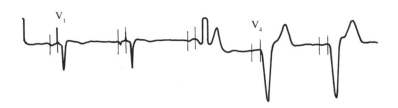

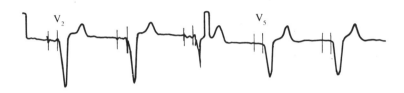

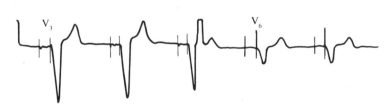

Chest leads   17.5 min/sec; 0.75 cm/mV

114 A 36-year-old woman, weighing 60 kg, is admitted following a suspected overdose. No tablets are found at gastric lavage and salicylate and paracetamol are not detected in the plasma. She is admitted for observation. Eleven hours after admission the patient's condition deteriorates and she rapidly becomes unconscious, with a respiratory rate of 36/minute. The following results are obtained:

Sodium	136 mmol/l
Potassium	5.7 mmol/l
Glucose	4.8 mmol/l
Bicarbonate (standardized)	8 mmol/l
Anion gap	36
Base excess	−20
Lactate	high
Urinalysis	crystalluria
PTT	15 s

a) What is the patient's calculated total bicarbonate (HCO_3^-) deficit?
b) What is the diagnosis? What further complications may occur?
c) What are the three principles of management?

115 The following results are obtained in a 27-year-old woman undergoing investigation for hypertension:

Sodium	136 mmol/l
Potassium	3.4 mmol/l
Urea	6.8 mmol/l
Creatinine	127 μmol/l
Right renal vein renin	× 1.5 inferior vena cava renin level
Left renal vein renin	× 2 inferior vena cava renin level

a) What is the probable diagnosis?
b) What is the explanation for the observed renin measurements?
c) What is the treatment of choice?
d) 36 hours following treatment, the patient's BP is 110/70 lying and 90/40 standing. How do you explain the postural hypotension observed 36 hours after therapy?

116 The following results are obtained during investigation of a 64-year-old patient with back pain, anaemia and an acute phase response.

Hb	9 g/dl
MCV	84 fl
WBC	$6.8 \times 10^9/l$
Platelets	$276 \times 10^9/l$
ESR	100 mm in the first hour
Sodium	138 mmol/l
Potassium	3.3 mmol/l
Urea	9.9 mmol/l
Creatinine	183 μmol/l
Bicarbonate	15 mmol/l
Chloride	109 mmol/l
Alkaline phosphatase	174 iu/l
Calcium (corrected)	2.8 mmol/l
Glucose	4.3 mmol/l
Urinalysis (early morning)	pH 5.2
	protein +++
	glucose ++

a) What is the diagnosis?
b) Why is the urine well acidified?
c) What diagnostic procedures are indicated?
d) What urine constituent is the likely cause of proteinuria?

117 A 65-year-old accountant presented to the Casualty Department complaining of acute swelling of both his legs. The swelling had not been present 7 days previously, but was now so severe that he could not put his trousers on to go to work. He had also noticed that his left testicle had enlarged gradually during the previous 2 months, but had been too embarrassed to mention this to his GP.

He was a very fit man, who walked for an hour on Hampstead Heath 4 times a week. He did not smoke, drank a glass of red wine every evening, and was married with 2 children at university. He had not visited any foreign countries, apart from a recent business trip to Orlando, USA 2 months prior to admission.

Examination showed an anxious thin man with marked oedema of the legs. The oedema pitted readily on digital pressure and involved both legs from just below the inguinal ligament to the dorsum of the feet. His pulse was 84 beats per minute, respiratory rate 17 per minute, and his JVP was 3 cm above the angle of Louis. Temperature was 38.8°C.

Urea and electrolytes were normal. FBC: Hb 17.8 g/dl, MCV 88 fl, WCC $8.6 \times 10^9/l$, platelets $421 \times 10^9/l$.

a) What is the likely diagnosis?
b) What investigations are required?

118 The following results were obtained in a patient with severe loin pain:

Sodium	138 mmol/l
Potassium	2.5 mmol/l
Urea	3.8 mmol/l
Chloride	114 mmol/l
Anion gap	12
Urinary pH	6.1

a) What is the bicarbonate concentration?
b) What is the diagnosis? What is the cause of the loin pain?

119 A 43-year-old depressed woman is admitted with an overdose. A number of different empty bottles of tablets are found in her bedroom, and it is not clear what she has taken. Aspirin or paracetamol seem the most likely possibilities.

a) What clinical features would suggest aspirin overdose?
b) What type of initial biochemical disturbance would be expected? How might this change?
c) Explain the mechanisms which produce the metabolic disturbances in this condition.
d) How do salicylate levels correlate with toxicity?
e) What is the treatment?

120 A 61-year-old female hospital domestic presented with an 8-week history of shivering attacks, increasing shortness of breath and leg oedema. Appetite was decreased and she had lost 3 kg in weight over this period. Past medical history included a perforated peptic ulcer 20 years previously and non-insulin-dependent diabetes mellitus. On admission she was taking glibenclamide 10 mg o.d. She was a non-smoker and drank 10 glasses of rum per week. Five months ago she returned from a 4-week visit to her birthplace on the island of St Lucia.

On examination she was pyrexial 37.8°C, clinically pale. Pulse 90 regular, BP 130/85 mmHg. Normal sclerae, no lymphadenopathy. Normal heart sounds with an apical systolic ejection murmur. Decreased movement on the right side of the chest with dull percussion note, diminished tactile vocal fremitus and absent breath sounds. The abdomen was soft with no organomegaly and the rest of the examination was normal.

Investigations:

Hb	9 g/dl
MCV	85 fl
Sickle cell	negative
WBC	8.9×10^9/l — 87% neutrophils
Platelets	450×10^9/l
ESR	66 mm in the first hour
Iron	6.0 µmol/l
Transferrin	1.5 g/l
Sodium	140 mmol/l
Potassium	4.5 mmol/l
Urea	5 mmol/l
Creatinine	130 µmol/l
Total protein	65 g/l
Albumin	19 g/l
Aspartate amino-transferase	45 iu/l
Bilirubin	15 µmol/l
Alkaline phosphatase	160 iu/l
PT	19.3 s
PTTK	43 s
Autoantibody screen	weak positive ANA
Blood cultures	*Streptococcus milleri*
Urine	normal
Chest X-ray	right pleural effusion
Pleural fluid	protein 62 g/l

a) What is the likely diagnosis and how would you confirm your diagnosis?
b) How would you manage the patient?

121 A 53-year-old hypertensive diabetic man presented to casualty feeling acutely dizzy and vomiting, with difficulty in speaking and a 'peculiar feeling' in his right arm and leg, and the left side of his face.
a) What is the probable diagnosis?
b) What physical signs would you expect to elicit?
c) i) Where is the lesion and ii) which vessel supplies this area?
d) How can the clinical findings be related directly to specific regions in the brain?

122 A 23-year-old woman attends her GP for contraceptive advice. Her blood pressure is found to be 158/98 mmHg and she has Grade I hypertensive retinal changes. One week later she is seen in a medical outpatients clinic. She has no personal or family history of note, and in particular no history of cardiac or renal disease. On direct questioning she admits to a 'viral illness' some weeks previously. She is not taking any prescribed or proprietary medications. On examination the registrar describes her appearance as 'thin and drawn', though she denies any weight loss. Her BP is 170/104 in both arms and there is no radiofemoral delay. The retinal changes are confirmed. There is no abdominal bruit. A Grade I ejection systolic murmur is noted at the base of the heart. The rest of the examination is normal.
    The following investigations are performed in outpatients:

Hb	11.5 g/dl
WBC	7.6×10^9/l
Platelets	376×10^9/l
Sodium	138 mmol/l
Potassium	4.4 mmol/l
Bicarbonate	22 mmol/l
Urea	11.5 mmol/l
Creatinine	156 μmol/l
Glucose	6.9 mmol/l
Urinalysis	blood ++, protein ++

MSU: 10^3 organisms mixed growth
Urine microscopy — 30 red cells/hpf, scanty granular casts
Antinuclear antibody — 1/80 homogeneous pattern
C3 17% NHP (N >60%)
C4 69% NHP (N >60%)
CH50 67% NHP (N >60%)
ECG and CXR are normal.
The patient is admitted for further investigation.

a) Suggest a likely diagnosis. What non-invasive investigation may support your clinical diagnosis?
b) Give a differential diagnosis.

123 Opposite is a series of excerpts from a 24 hour tape (lead V1).
a) What is demonstrated?

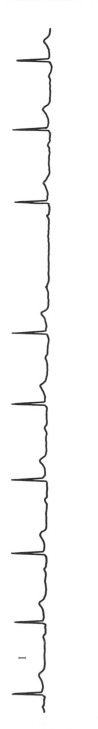

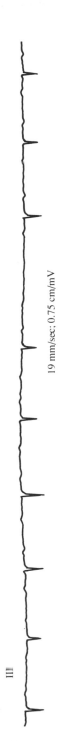

19 mm/sec; 0.75 cm/mV

124 This is a routine ECG.
    a) What is the predominant rhythm in the 12 lead recordings?
    b) In the rhythm strip, is atrial depolarization normal?

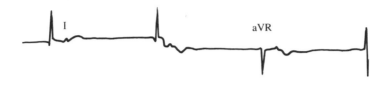

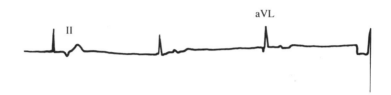

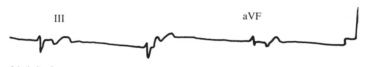

Limb leads

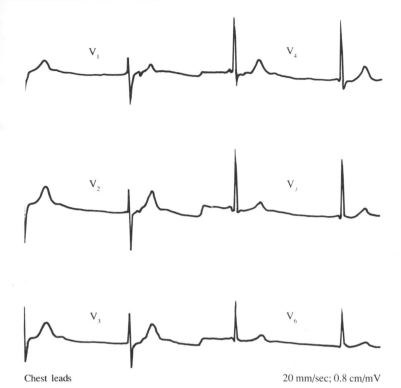

V₁   V₄

V₂   V₃

V₃   V₆

Chest leads   20 mm/sec; 0.8 cm/mV

125 A 63-year-old man came into A&E with a 2-day history of severe leg pains, and increasing difficulty in walking. He was previously well, but both he and his wife had 'flu 10 days earlier. On examination, he was apyrexial, pulse 90 SR, BP 120/70 mmHg, chest clear, RR 22; no neck stiffness, but both his arms and legs were weak, and no tendon reflexes could be elicited.

a) What is the diagnosis?
b) What investigation is required? What would the findings be? Give a differential diagnosis of these findings.
c) What are the principles of management?
d) Name two related neurological conditions.

126 A 28-year-old asthmatic man is admitted from outpatients with a 3-week history of progressive lower limb swelling. The rest of his history is unremarkable and his only medications are a Ventolin inhaler, and a proprietary analgesic for a sporting injury sustained 5 weeks previously.

Examination confirms pitting oedema to the thighs. Blood pressure is 130/78 with no postural hypotension.

The following investigations are performed:

Sodium	139 mmol/l
Potassium	4.8 mmol/l
Urea	8.7 mmol/l
Creatinine	112 µmol/l
Albumin	22 g/l
Urinalysis	protein ++++, blood negative
24-hr urine protein	5.7 g

Renal biopsy — normal appearances on light microscopy, podocyte effacement on electron microscopy.

The patient's weight on admission is 83 kg. His fluid intake is restricted to 1 litre per day, he is given a low-salt diet, and is prescribed a loop diuretic and high-dose steroids. Eight days later his weight is 71 kg and his serum urea and creatinine are 32 and 170 respectively. Urinalysis shows 4+ proteinuria and 3+ of blood. He informs the nursing staff of bilateral loin ache. That afternoon he experiences a sudden onset of shortness of breath, and arterial blood gas analysis shows a pO_2 of 6.7 kPa and a pCO_2 of 3.3 kPa.

a) What is the initial diagnosis? Give two potential causes of the initial renal lesion.

b) What complication has occurred?

127 A 27-year-old man is admitted to casualty very pale and unwell. He has a history of 2–3 weeks' haemoptysis and increasing malaise, and during the 24 hours prior to admission he has noticed a fall in urine output, and blood in his urine.

On examination: pulse 130 sinus rhythm; BP 145/95 mmHg; JVP + 9cm; RR 24/min; scattered crackles in both lung fields on auscultation.

Investigations:

Hb	8.3 g/dl mildly hypochromic
WBC	$11.8 \times 10^9/l$
Platelets	$621 \times 10^9/l$
Clotting	normal
Sodium	136 mmol/l
Potassium	7.6 mmol/l
Urea	32.1 mmol/l
Creatinine	769 µmol/l
ECG	peaked T-waves
CXR	patchy interstitial shadowing both lungs
Urine dipstick	protein +++, blood +++

a) What is the likely diagnosis? What other questions would you ask?
b) What other tests should be performed urgently?
c) What is the immediate priority in this patient's management?

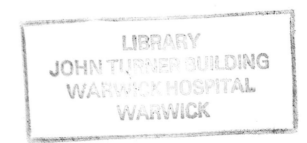

128 A A 45-year-old man presented to the rheumatology clinic with painful knees. Past medical history included meningococcal meningitis at the age of 20 and gonorrhoea at the age of 24. He had otherwise enjoyed good health until 2 years ago when he became impotent and this had led to marital difficulties. He smoked 20 cigarettes a day and drank 4 pints of beer per night when on leave in the United Kingdom.

On examination he looked well with a marked suntan, having recently returned from Saudi Arabia where he worked as an engineer. Marked crepitus was present in both knees. Testes were small and pubic hair sparse.

Investigations:

Hb	14 g/dl
WBC	$5 \times 10^9/l$
ESR	15 mm in the first hour
Urea and electrolytes	normal
Urine dipstick	glucose ++

a) What is the cause of the arthritis? What is the likely diagnosis?
b) How would you confirm your diagnosis?

B A 57-year-old woman is admitted following a collapse. She complains of recent difficulty in rising from her armchair. Her blood pressure is 168/108 with 8 mmHg systolic postural drop. She has recently been taking a proprietary analgesic for osteoarthritis. The following results are obtained:

Sodium	136 mmol/l
Potassium	6.8 mmol/l
Bicarbonate	16 mmol/l
Urea	17 mmol/l
Creatinine	270 µmol/l
Chloride	110 mmol/l
HbA1c	9%
Aldosterone	low
Urinalysis	protein +++

a) What is the underlying diagnosis?
b) What is the serum renin concentration likely to be?
c) What is the likely explanation for the collapse?
d) Give two possible causes of the lower limb weakness.

129 A 39-year-old aerobics instructor presents with a 3-month history of increasing weight and abdominal girth. She is very diet-conscious and despite reducing her caloric intake and continuing to exercise regularly she has put on 3 kg in weight during the previous 2 months. She does not smoke, or abuse alcohol. She complains of profound tiredness and malaise, and is unable to keep up with the advanced aerobics class. Further history of note is that her mother died of breast cancer around the age of 45.

On examination she is a thin-looking woman, with no jaundice, cyanosis or anaemia. Jugular venous pressure is 2 cm above the manubriosternal angle, and her abdomen is prominent. Her cardiac, respiratory and abdominal examination are normal. Breast examination is normal, and there is no peripheral oedema.

a) What is the likely diagnosis? Give three possible causes of this clinical picture.

b) What investigations should be performed?

130 A 45-year-old farmer from a remote rural village in Wales is visiting his relatives in London. He consumes 8 pints of beer per day, smokes 30 cigarettes a day, and also takes a proprietary analgesic on a regular basis for morning headaches. He presents to casualty with three episodes of frank haematemesis, and one episode of melaena.

On examination the patient is obese, clinically pale but not jaundiced. He does have a small amount of ascites, and four spider naevi on his chest. He has mild hyperinflation of both lungs. Blood pressure is 110/80 supine, and 90/60 sitting. His pulse is 106 beats per minute. Emergency blood tests demonstrate a haemoglobin of 12 g/dl, WBC 14.6×10^9/l, platelets 236×10^9/l; urea 2 mmol/l, creatinine 112 μmol/l.

The locum surgical specialist registrar does an emergency gastroscopy with you in casualty. The procedure is well tolerated, and he reports three very large varices 7 cm from the gastro-oesophageal junction, and copious fresh blood in the stomach. Having confirmed his clinical diagnosis the registrar expresses his desire to terminate the procedure.

a) What advice would you offer the surgical specialist registrar?

b) What therapy should be initiated?

131 A young woman presents with intermittent ankle swelling and abdominal pain, and on two occasions has attended Accident and Emergency with swelling of the neck. She is a keen gardener, takes macrolide antibiotics on a regular basis for troublesome upper respiratory tract infections, and is allergic to penicillin. When she attended previously with neck swelling she was treated with adrenalin and hydrocortisone with little immediate benefit.

Investigations performed at the time of an acute attack revealed normal haemoglobin, and a white cell count of 10.1 × 10^9/l. Throat swab showed *Candida albicans*. C4 levels measured on two occasions at time of presentation of acute attacks were 0.08 mg/l and 0.07 mg/l (normal >0.15 mg/l). C1 esterase inhibitor levels measured in the local laboratory were normal on two occasions.

a) What is the likely diagnosis, and how would you confirm this?
b) What treatment would you recommend should the patient present to casualty with a further attack?
c) What other advice would you give the patient?

132 A 59-year-old patient with an alcohol intake of 6 units per day presents with tiredness, jaundice, and a change in bowel habit. He has lost 4 kg over 3 months.

On examination he is cachectic, his fingers are deeply stained from smoking, and he is severely jaundiced. Chest examination reveals hyperinflation, with inspiratory crepitations. Jugular venous pressure is normal. Cardiac auscultation reveals soft first and second heart sounds, with no accessory sounds. There is no peripheral oedema. Abdominal examination demonstrates no ascites or organomegaly.

Blood tests are as follows:
Urea and electrolytes normal
Liver function tests: ALT 40 iu/l; AST 45 iu/l, albumin 35 g/l, bilirubin 110 μmol/l
Full blood count: Hb 11 g/dl, MCV 72 fl, platelets 156 × 10^9/l, WCC 8.7 × 10^9/l.

a) What two conditions may explain his jaundice, and which of the blood tests reported above will help to discriminate between the two?
b) What two radiological examinations will confirm the diagnosis?

133 A 36-year-old, previously fit solicitor is brought into the A&E department with vomiting and acute shortness of breath. She was hypertensive in the last trimesters of her two pregnancies. She is a non-smoker, and drinks in moderation. She has a history of frequent migraines, and mild Raynaud's phenomenon. She has just returned from a 2-week holiday in the Dordogne, where she stayed in a local farmhouse. She complained of diarrhoea and abdominal pain in the week prior to admission. The other members of the family experienced a mild and self-limiting gastroenteritis while on holiday.

She looks acutely unwell with a respiratory rate of 34, temperature 37.8°C and a pulse of 120 beats per minute. JVP is 4 cm above the sternal notch. Blood pressure is 140/90, chest clear, abdomen soft and non-tender. The patient's cardiac monitor shows multiple ventricular ectopic beats. Blood gases demonstrate a pH of 7.03, and a pO_2 of 8.3 kPa on air, pCO_2 of 1.7 kPa, and a bicarbonate of 14 mmol/l. Blood glucose is 5.7 mmol/l. Ketones are not demonstrated in the urine, but ++ blood and + protein are detected.

a) What urgent investigations would you perform?
b) What is the likely diagnosis?
c) How would you manage this patient in the first 48 hours of her hospital stay?
d) What advice would you provide for family and carers?

134 A 48-year-old pathologist presents with a 3-month history of tiredness, weight loss of 1.5 kg, myalgia, and intermittent pain and swelling of both calves and forearms. The swelling is associated with tingling in the thumb and first finger of the hand, and fluctuating erythema affecting the anterior surface of the forearm. The patient had recorded temperatures of 38°C on several occasions. The patient was Hungarian, and visited his native country 3 to 4 times per year; he had recently spent a holiday in his lakeside villa in the mountainous region of Hungary.

Baseline investigations performed by his GP showed Hb of 11.4 g/dl, platelet count $157 \times 10^9/l$, total WCC of $11.1 \times 10^9/l$, 40% eosinophils. Urea and electrolytes and liver function tests were normal.

a) Give a differential diagnosis. What is the most likely diagnosis? What other investigations would you perform?
b) Is there any other specific information you would seek in the history?

135 A 62-year-old retired female nursery school teacher was referred to medical outpatients department with progressive visual impairment, ankle oedema, and ulceration of skin nodules over her elbows. She also had increasingly painful second and third digits of the left hand, with painful ulcerating lesions of the finger pulps of these digits.

She had a 14-year history of disabling rheumatoid arthritis with nodulosis and had been treated for 11 years with oral prednisolone at a dose of between 7.5 and 25 mg daily. Urinalysis revealed 4+ proteinuria; the patient's serum albumin was 24 g/l, and creatinine 234 mmol/l.

a) What specific features would you look for on examination of this patient?
b) What are the two likely diagnoses?
c) What further investigations would you perform?
d) How would you manage this patient?

136 A 42-year-old single male presents with a history of breathlessness of acute onset. The patient works as a sales manager for a motor spares accessories firm, and travels extensively in Eastern Europe.

On examination he looks thin, and has lost weight. His respiratory rate is 22 per minute, with no abnormal signs on clinical examination of the chest. His temperature is 38.2°C and pulse 104 beats per minute. He had attended casualty the previous day, and a blood count was performed. Hb was 11.3 g/dl, normochromic normocytic, WCC 2.7×10^9/l, platelets 110×10^9/l, urea and electrolytes normal.

On his second admission an emergency AP chest X-ray was performed which showed a 15% pneumothorax on the left, and possible left midzone consolidation.

a) What further investigations would you perform?
b) What is the likely diagnosis, and what other possibilities would you consider?
c) How would you manage this patient?

137 A 27-year-old student teacher presents with joint pains, affecting the small joints of the hands, shoulders and both knees. These came on acutely, but during the previous 2 weeks the patient had had a short-lived illness characterized by an evanescent rash and 2 days of diarrhoea.

On examination the patient had an effusion of the left knee, and synovitis of the second and third metacarpophalangeal joints of both hands, and pain on flexion of the wrists of both hands.

Investigations:

HB 10.9 g/dl, platelets 143 × 10⁹/l, WCC 4.8 × 10⁹/l.
Biochemical profile: normal.
Rheumatoid factor positive 1/20, ANA negative, anticardiolipin IgG 43.6 AEU (normal range <10), anticardiolipin IgM 26.3 AEU (normal <9).

a) What is the likely diagnosis?
b) What is the main differential?
c) What specific blood tests will you perform?

138 A 63-year-old woman, with a long history of incapacitating migrainous headaches and hypertension, presents with confusion and left loin pain. On examination she is tender in the left loin, pulse of 97 per minute, temperature of 38.5°C. Urinalysis reveals 1 + proteinuria with no haematuria. Further investigation confirms Na⁺ 136 mmol/l, K⁺ 5.1 mmol/l, urea 41.6 mmol/l, creatinine 837 μmol/l.

a) What is the nature of the presenting problem? What is the most likely underlying diagnosis?
b) What radiological investigation should be performed acutely?
c) What emergency treatment is required?
d) What further radiological investigation may be indicated to confirm the diagnosis?
e) How would you manage this patient's fluid balance during the next 24 hours?

139 A 24-year-old professional squash player collapses on the court during an exhibition match. You are in the audience and are called to resuscitate him. You perform cardiopulmonary resuscitation, and when the ambulance arrives defibrillation leads to a return of sinus rhythm, and restoration of blood pressure.

a) Name two underlying cardiac conditions which could explain this presentation.

b) What common cerebral condition can present with sudden death in patients in this age group?

c) The patient's wife tells you that he had recently been self-medicating for hay fever. How may this be relevant to his presentation?

140 A 34-year-old woman presented with shortness of breath, which had become worse during the past year. She also complained of a non-productive cough. She had two children aged 7 and 10 who were well. She was a heavy smoker, and used 4 units of alcohol per day. The patient also used non-steroidal anti-inflammatory drugs and paracetamol on a daily basis for minor aches and pains and headaches. She had a 10-year history of recurrent urinary tract infections.

On examination she had a respiratory rate of 34 per minute, with end-inspiratory crackles audible over both lung bases. During exercise, cyanosis developed.

a) What investigations will you do?

b) What is the most likely diagnosis?

c) What is the prognosis in this patient?

141 A 45-year-old refugee from Equatorial Africa presents to the casualty department with abdominal pain, jaundice, and anorexia. Her symptoms started 10 days prior to presentation. She has been resident in the UK for 2 months, and has been previously well. There is no history of exposure to others with jaundice, and nobody in her extended family has these symptoms.

On examination she is tender over the right hypochondrium. The liver is not enlarged. Her sclerae are yellow, and she is not anaemic. The rest of the examination, including vaginal and rectal examination, is normal.

Hepatitis B and C serology performed by her general practitioner 7 days prior to presentation are negative. IgG antibodies to Hepatitis A and EBV were detectable in serum. The general practitioner also performed liver function tests which demonstrated a raised AST (95 iu/l), a bilirubin of 93 μmol/l and a raised alkaline phosphatase (395 iu/l). Full blood count demonstrated the following: Hb 12.1 g/dl, WCC 14.2 × 10⁹/l, neutrophils 7.7 × 10⁹/l, lymphocytes 3.4 × 10⁹/l, eosinophils 2.2 × 10⁹/l.

a) Suggest a likely diagnosis.
b) What investigations will you perform?
c) What therapy will you recommend?

142 A 54-year-old Indian man presented to a medical outpatients department with a 2-year history of severe abdominal pain. The pain occurred twice a month, and was not precipitated by any specific event. There was also no relation to food or passage of stool. The patient complained of generalized mild arthralgia, for which he had been taking a remedy provided by the local Indian pharmacy. He had been previously investigated as an in-patient under care of the gastroenterology firm. A colonoscopic examination was normal, as was a gastroscopy.

The notes from this admission demonstrated that during a 3-day period he remained afebrile, his urea and electrolytes were abnormal, as were liver function tests, but a microcytic anaemia was noted. Stool and urine porphyrins, blood glucose, and HbA1C were normal. Stool culture negative. His pain subsided after one day in hospital and he was discharged with no diagnosis.

On examination in the clinic the patient was noted to have weakness of wrist extension on the right, but no sensory deficit, and had widespread osteoarthritis, affecting the small joints of the hands, knees and hips.

a) What is the likely diagnosis?
b) Give three tests which you would perform.
c) What is the treatment?

143 A 56-year-old man treated for mycobacterial tuberculosis for 9 months complains of numb feet. Nerve conduction studies show the following:

Neural sensory action potential 8 μV (normal >15 μV)
Median nerve sensory action potential 4 μV (normal > 20 μV)
Common peroneal motor nerve velocity 48 m/s (normal >45 m/s)

a) What type of neuropathy is present? What is the likely explanation in this patient?
b) Give three other recognized causes of this type of neuropathy.

144 A 45-year-old man is referred urgently by his GP with a clinical diagnosis of left lower pneumonia, in association with a high fever, and breathlessness. In the past the patient had undergone a renal transplant for Alport's syndrome at the age of 33 years. He had had two attacks of gout during the previous 6 weeks, and had been started on prophylactic treatment by the local rheumatologist.

   Clinical examination confirms the general practitioner's diagnosis, and a CXR shows extensive left basal consolidation. Blood tests, performed urgently in A&E, reveal the following:

Hb	15 g/dl
WBC	0.7 × 10⁹/l
Platelets	233 × 10⁹/l
Sodium	136 mmol/l
Potassium	4 mmol/l
Urea	12 mmol/l
Creatinine	167 μmol/l
Bicarbonate	20 mmol/l
Calcium	2.4 mmol/l
Phosphate	1.0 mmol/l.

a) What is the likely explanation for the clinical picture? What other history would you endeavour to obtain from the patient?
b) How would you manage this patient?

145 A 25-year-old male complained of muscle cramps which prevented him from playing football. He had always experienced muscle pain during the initial period of exercise but found that his symptoms passed off with continued graduated exertion. He was otherwise fit and well and there was no relevant family history. General examination was unremarkable and neurologically he had no evidence of muscle weakness.

Baseline investigations including muscle enzymes and an EMG were normal. An Ischaemic Forearm test was performed which demonstrated no rise in the venous lactate level after cessation of exercise.

a) What is the likely diagnosis?
b) How would you confirm this?

146 A 56-year-old woman presents to medical OPD with a 4-month history of increasing exertional breathlessness and vague chest pain. She describes having a 'blackout' while walking up a cliff path on a recent holiday. She has been treated for mild 'asthma' for 4 years by her GP and has troublesome osteoarthritis of both hips, thought to be secondary to moderate obesity when younger.

On examination, the patient weighs 54 kg, and is 5'8" in height. Cardiovascular examination reveals a sinus tachycardia, an accentuated pulmonary second heart sound, and a cardiac thrust palpable along the left sternal border. The respiratory rate is elevated at 24/minute, but breath sounds are entirely normal throughout both lung fields. PEFR is within the normal range for age and body mass.

a) What is the likely diagnosis?
b) What other information should be sought in the history?
c) How would you investigate this patient?

147 A 26-year-old solicitor undergoes a private 'health screen' before taking up a new job. The screening involves a range of blood tests, subsequent to which referral to medical outpatients is recommended. In the referral letter to the clinic, the following results are available:

Calcium	2.95 mmol/l
Serum magnesium	1.02 mmol/l (marginally elevated)
Phosphate	1.3 mmol/l
24-hour urinary calcium excretion	2.1 mmol.

The patient is entirely well, but tells you that his mother had an operation on her neck in middle age because she was noted to have a high blood calcium.

a) What is the likely diagnosis? Which tests specifically support this?
b) What further investigations may be informative?
c) How would you manage this patient?

148 A 22-year-old Caucasian girl was referred to Rheumatology by her GP. She had had a sore throat 10 days previously, which was treated with Erythromycin, of which she only took 3 days' treatment.

Presenting complaint was of pain in both buttocks, with radiation in a sciatic distribution on the right. She was systemically well, but felt that the pain was getting worse, and she had taken 6 dihydrocodeine tablets during the previous 12 hours. Her GP had performed some blood test 2 days before, which showed:

Hb	9.7 g/dl
Platelets	673×10^9/l
WBC	31.6×10^9/l
ESR	119 mm in the first hour
CRP	236 mg/l
Biochemical profile	normal.

On examination, both buttocks were tender; there was no lymphadenopathy; temperature 37°C; pulse 92 bpm; BP 100/60; neither neck stiffness or neurological deficit was detected.
The patient was admitted. Over the next 36 hours the patient became febrile (40°C) and toxic. Her pain increased and her CRP rose to 397 mg/l.

a) Is there anything else you would ask about in the history?
b) What investigations would you perform?
c) What treatment would you initiate?
d) Give a differential diagnosis. What is the most likely diagnosis?
e) What is the prognosis in this condition?

Answers

1 **a) Fasting hypoglycaemia** due to excess insulin secretion. With a blood glucose of 2.9 mmol/l, plasma insulin level should be <3 mU/l.

b) An insulinoma is the commonest cause of excess insulin secretion. The important differential diagnosis in this case is self-administration of insulin. The latter can be excluded by measurement of plasma-immunoreactive C-peptide which will be low in cases of exogenous insulin administration and high with an endogenous insulin source. Retroperitoneal fibrosarcoma and mesothelioma can also induce hypoglycaemia by secretion of insulin-like growth factors.

Spontaneous hypoglycaemia can be divided into 2 groups:
1) Fasting hypoglycaemia — symptoms occur at night, in the early morning or after a fast. This group can be subdivided into

i) Excess insulin production or self-administration (no ketosis), e.g.
   Insulinoma
   Retroperitoneal fibrosarcoma
   Mesothelioma
ii) Non-insulin induced causes (ketonaemia is a feature) e.g.
   Liver failure
   Addison's disease, hypopituitarism
   Ethanol, sulphonylureas, aspirin, propranolol
   Septicaemia, malaria
   Autoimmune hypoglycaemia — insulin receptor autoantibodies
   End-stage renal disease

2) Post-prandial or reactive hypoglycaemia — symptoms occur 2–4 hours after eating.

Insulinoma
One of the commonest causes of non-diabetic fasting-induced hypoglycaemia. These are tumours of the B cells and can occur in any part of the pancreas. The majority are benign and slow growing, but 10% are malignant.
   Median age of presentation is the 5th decade. Patients typically present with drowsiness on waking which is relieved by eating. Other modes of presentation include fits, dizziness, diplopia and paraesthesiae. Patients may become obese as their calorie consumption increases in an attempt to avoid symptoms.

2 **a)** Ischaemic heart disease is the commonest cause of atrial arrhythmias.

b) Insertion of a pacemaker. Whatever the atrial rhythm there is atrioventricular (AV) nodal dysfunction with AV conduction disturbance.

c) Quinidine speeds the conduction through the AV node and can cause 1:1 conduction of atrial flutter with a ventricular rate of 300.

3 a) i) Reversible obstructive airways disease — presumably an infective exacerbation of asthma in this case. ii) (Variable) extrathoracic tracheal obstruction.
Note: C is a normal flow–volume loop.

The first flow–volume loop in the question is typical of severe obstructive airways disease. The normal expiratory limb in the second loop confirms that this must be reversible airways obstruction, i.e. asthma. The inspiratory limb of the second flow loop is abnormal. The MIF_{50} is the inspiratory flow rate at 50% of the vital capacity and in this instance is approximately half that expected. This confirms an extrathoracic tracheal obstruction which must be variable as the expiratory limb is unaffected. In the clinical context, this is likely to be a consequence of long-term intubation, with development of a tracheal stricture — this patient should have been managed with a tracheostomy. Other causes of extrathoracic tracheal obstruction include vocal cord palsies, malignancy and infective and inflammatory conditions, including Wegener's granulomatosis and syphilis. The other important pattern of flow–volume loop is that of a fixed intrathoracic tracheal obstruction, for example due to hilar malignancy, and in this instance both the inspiratory and expiratory limbs will be flattened.

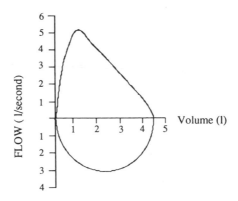

4 a) The most likely diagnosis is **acute rheumatic fever** and a **recent hepatitis A infection.**

b) Immediate management is bed rest, physiotherapy and acetyl-salicylate as an anti-inflammatory agent (6–12 g/day) to achieve blood levels between 2.1 and 2.4 mmol/l. The dramatic response of the arthritis to salicylate therapy is characteristic. Oral penicillin 125–250 mg 12-hourly should be taken until the age of 20 years in all patients who have had carditis, to decrease the risk of a further attack of rheumatic fever. Daily oral penicillin or monthly intramuscular penicillin should be continued in adults who continue to be exposed to young children. There is no evidence that salicylates or steroids influence the prognosis.

She fulfils the **Duckett–Jones criteria** for acute rheumatic fever, i.e. two major criteria or one major and two minor criteria plus evidence of a recent streptococcal infection.

Major criteria of rheumatic fever include polyarthritis, carditis, erythema marginatum, subcutaneous nodules (Aschoff) and chorea.

Minor criteria include previous rheumatic fever, fever, arthralgia, raised ESR and prolonged P–R interval.

Evidence of recent group A streptococcal infection includes i) isolation of haemolytic streptococci from a throat swab, ii) rising antibody titre and iii) recent scarlet fever.

The differential diagnosis of rheumatic fever includes:
1) Rubella
2) Still's disease — childhood onset rheumatoid arthritis
3) Hepatitis
4) Infective endocarditis
5) Sickle cell disease
6) Gonococcal arthritis
7) Malignancy — leukaemia or lymphoma
8) Familial Mediterranean Fever.

The infectious hepatitis A acquired in Pakistan had settled before the onset of this illness (note there is no significant change in the hepatitis A antibody titres). The raised AST is caused by the rheumatic fever and the elevation of the enzyme is a measure of the severity of the attack.

5 A

a) The diagnosis is **pyschogenic polydipsia** (high 24-hour urine volumes). She is normovolaemic, as assessed by physical examination, and is hypotonic and hyponatraemic. This can only be caused by excess water in the extracellular space. The possibilities are ADH-dependent water retention, ADH-independent water retention (e.g. in chronic renal failure) or excess water intake. In the case of neurogenic diabetes insipidus the plasma osmolality and sodium are usually normal provided water is freely available.

b) In psychogenic polydipsia the ADH is appropriately low. If there is difficulty in distinguishing between neurogenic diabetes insipidus and psychogenic polydipsia, a water deprivation test should be performed with serial measurement of weight, plasma and urine osmolality and plasma ADH. The plasma osmolality should rise to above 290 mmol/l (to ensure an adequate stimulus for ADH secretion); in the case of true diabetes insipidus the urine osmolality will not increase appropriately. Desmopressin (an analogue of ADH) is then given; a rise in the osmolality of the urine will be seen with neurogenic diabetes insipidus but not with nephrogenic diabetes insipidus. In nephrogenic diabetes insipidus there is end-organ resistance to ADH (ADH levels typically normal). In some cases of psychogenic polydipsia the results of the water deprivation test may be difficult to interpret. This may be resolved by an infusion of hypertonic saline with serial measurements of plasma and urine osmolalities, along with plasma ADH levels and urine volumes.

B

a) Suprapubic bladder aspiration.

The urine sample contains numerous epithelial cells and a mixed-bacterial flora of oral commensals, strongly suggesting that the urine had been contaminated. On detailed examination of the mucosal cavity a laceration was seen on the inside of the cheek. The patient admitted that the injury was self-inflicted and that he had been spitting blood into his urine.

6 A

a) Hypocalcaemia leads to increased neuromuscular excitability, resulting in paraesthesiae of the extremities and circumoral areas, tetany, muscle cramps and fits.

Chvostek's test — tapping the facial nerve — may elicit a twitch.

Trousseau's sign — inflation of a sphygmomanometer cuff for 3 minutes above the diastolic pressure may elicit carpopedal spasm.

b) Hypomagnesaemia subsequent to *cis*-platinum therapy. Hypomagnesaemia occurs in approximately 50% of patients treated with *cis*-platinum as a result of renal magnesium loss. Hypomagnesaemia results in hypocalcaemia due to inhibition of parathyroid hormone release and impaired end-organ response to parathyroid hormone.

The patient should be given intravenous magnesium sulphate until magnesium levels normalize.

B

a) Congestive cardiac failure.

b) The biochemical picture of low serum sodium, low potassium, high bicarbonate and elevated urea is explained by the secondary hypoaldosteronism that complicates severe congestive cardiac failure. Note that although serum sodium levels are low, total body serum sodium levels are high. The hypoalbuminaemia is explained by the protein-losing enteropathy which may complicate such a picture with a grossly oedematous intestinal mucosa. Oral drugs are often ineffective in such cases due to decreased absorption, and drugs need to be given intravenously.

7 a) i) Recurrent lymphoma
    ii) Opportunistic infection — patient is immunosuppressed (particularly with *Pneumocystis carinii*)
    iii) Hepatic abscess
  b) i) Bronchoscopy with washings and transbronchial biopsy
    ii) Ultrasound or CT scan of abdomen
    iii) Liver biopsy

Hodgkin's disease (Thomas Hodgkin 1832) is commoner overall in males, with two age peaks from 15–25 and 55–75 years of age. The disease is characterized by the presence of Reed–Sternberg cells. Four histological variants are described: i) lymphocyte predominant (10–15% — overall, have the best prognosis); ii) mixed cellularity (20–40%); iii) lymphocyte depleted (5–15%), and iv) nodular sclerosing (20–50%). Clinically, patients present with enlarged lymph nodes (usually neck or axilla) or a mediastinal mass on chest X-ray. 25% of patients have constitutional or B symptoms of pruritus, fever, alcohol-induced pain and >10% weight loss. Staging is according to the Ann Arbor classification — Stage I: A single lymph node or a single extralymphatic organ or site. Stage II: 2 or more lymph node regions or an extranodal site and lymph nodes, on the same side of the diaphragm. Stage III: Nodes on both sides of the diaphragm, with or without splenic involvement. Stage IV: Diffuse involvement of one or more extralymphatic sites, with or without lymphadenopathy.

Treatment, broadly, is mantle or inverted Y radiotherapy for Stages I and II disease (unless bulky). Stage III and IV disease, along with bulky stage II disease, are treated with combination chemotherapy using four drugs — the usual first choice being LOPP (chlorambucil, vincristine, procarbazine and prednisolone). Five-year survival without treatment is 10%; now it is 70–80% for all stages. Early stage, youth, the absence of B symptoms and good prognostic histology bode best.

The disease caused by *Pneumocystis carinii* is an extensive pneumonitis found almost exclusively in the immunosuppressed or immunodeficient host. Pathologically the disease is characterized by an extensive desquamative alveolitis. The organisms are clustered in the alveolar lumen. The 'foamy exudate' formerly described represents unstained clusters of cysts and alveolar cells with cytoplasmic vacuoles.

Clinical features include marked tachypnoea, dry cough and fever. Hypoxia is often marked and precedes radiological change. The typical X-ray shows diffuse, bilateral alveolar disease originating at the hilum and progressing peripherally.

For a definitive diagnosis *P. carinii* must be identified in lung tissue by fibreoptic bronchoscopy or open lung biopsy. Treatment is with either i) Trimethoprim-sulphamethoxazole (co-trimoxazole) or ii) pentamidine isothionate. Untreated, the fatality rate approaches 100%, but is reduced to 25% with one of these agents. Up to 15% of patients who recover will have a second episode. Chemoprophylaxis for high-risk patients is with co-trimoxazole, which is dependable for only as long as the drug is taken.

8 a) **A Meckel's diverticulum presenting with haemorrhage.**
The differential diagnosis includes Peutz–Jeghers syndrome,
hereditary haemorrhagic telangiectasia, Crohn's disease and
Familial Polyposis Coli, but the normal appearance of perioral
and perianal skin, oral mucosa and rectal mucosa make them
unlikely candidates.

A Meckel's diverticulum represents the remains of the vitello-
intestinal tract. It occurs in 2% of the population and is
approximately 2 cm in length and situated 2 ft from the ileocaecal
valve attached to the antimesenteric border. Heterotropic gastric
mucosa and pancreatic tissue are occasionally found in the
diverticulum.

The majority of patients are asymptomatic but recognized
complications include: inflammation — symptoms and signs
mimic appendicitis, intestinal obstruction and haemorrhage.
Bleeding occurs from adjacent small intestine mucosa when
ectopic gastric mucosa is present, and an acute bleed usually
manifests as the passage of bright red rectal blood. Alternatively
low grade blood loss may occur and complicate chronic peptic
ulceration. Clinically any child with painless rectal bleeding
should be assumed to have a Meckel's diverticulum.

b) Arteriography is of value in defining the site of bleeding when
blood loss exceeds 1 ml/min. Alternatively abdominal scanning
following injection of isotope-labelled red blood cells may help in
localizing the site of blood loss.

Technetium-99m scanning has a role in outlining ectopic
gastric mucosa as the isotope is concentrated in gastric mucosa.
Laparotomy is often necessary not only to confirm the diagnosis,
but also to provide definitive treatment.

9 a) **Hypergastrinaemia resulting in recurrent peptic
ulceration**. Up to 80% of patients develop a varying degree of
steatorrhoea following partial gastrectomy.

The fall in serum gastrin levels during the secretin test in a
patient who has undergone a Polya gastrectomy is highly
suggestive of **retained gastric antrum**. In contrast the gastrin
level in cases of a gastrin-secreting tumour (Zollinger–Ellison
syndrome) rises during the secretin test. In normal individuals
gastrin levels fall during the test.

b) The diagnosis of retained gastric antrum should be confirmed
at laparotomy.

10 a) Chronic hepatitis B-induced hepatitis, possibly acquired during childhood. The factors which determine whether a hepatitis B infection becomes chronic or full recovery occurs are not known. Ten percent of patients after an acute infection develop one of three chronic syndromes: i) normal histology but a chronic carrier; ii) chronic persistent hepatitis; iii) chronic active hepatitis which may progress to cirrhosis and is an important risk for the development of primary hepatocellular carcinoma. During the first years of chronic infection, virus replication is high; patients are HBs Ag and HBe Ag-positive but are e antibody-negative and are highly infectious. Later, patients develop antibodies to first HBc Ag then HBe Ag and finally HBs Ag. After many years HBs Ag and HBe Ag may be undetectable, although antibodies to the core protein (HBc Ag) remain detectable.

b) Investigations: i) HBe Ag, HBc antibody and HBs antibody to assess the patient's infectivity and immune response to the virus; ii) a liver biopsy and liver ultrasound to assess hepatic damage and any continuing liver inflammation or cirrhosis.

c) Indications for therapy include: i) infectivity, e.g. HBe Ag-positive patients, and ii) evidence of progressive liver disease (chronic active hepatitis). Decompensated cirrhosis is a contraindication. Treatment with antiviral agents and possibly interferon is useful even if the virus has become integrated into the host genome; improvement of the inflammatory liver disease will occur if viral replication is inhibited.

11 a) This man has spinal cord compression with nerve root involvement resulting in a sensory level at T10 and evidence of both pyramidical weakness and dorsal column involvement. Rectal tone is often preserved until late in spinal cord compression.

Radiology shows destruction of T8 and T9 vertebrae. The main differential diagnosis is between a malignant and an infectious process. Involvement of two adjacent vertebrae and loss of the disc space strongly suggests infection rather than malignancy. Night sweats which resolved after antibiotic therapy are a further clue. The lack of an acute phase response and normal white blood count do not favour malignancy. Spinal osteomyelitis may be associated with little systemic upset and furthermore he had received antibiotics. The change in bowel habit is solely the result of opiate analgesia.

Note: Back pain which radiates in a dermatomal distribution suggests nerve root involvement and therefore a disease process which involves the epidural space. The radiological appearance may lag behind the clinical disease by weeks or months.

b) CT scanning or MRI scanning. Isotope bone scans are helpful only when the plain X-rays are normal.

The treatment of spinal cord compression is urgent decompression, and the prognosis is related to the speed of diagnosis, as decompression, to be successful, must be undertaken early. There are two mechanisms causing neurological damage:

i) the formation of an epidural abscess with a mass effect, and
ii) thrombosis of the spinal arteries.

The treatment of spinal osteomyelitis is intravenous antibiotics for 6 weeks. Accurate microbiological diagnosis is essential and may be obtained by guided biopsy, if surgery is not required for spinal decompression.

The main organisms implicated in spinal osteomyelitis are *Staphylococcus aureus* (60%), enterobacteria (30%), acid-fast bacilli, brucella, *Haemophilus influenzae*, nocardia, candida, and *Treponema pallidum*. Organisms usually spread via the blood stream but direct invasion may occur, e.g. from a pharyngeal abscess.

12 a) Bartter's syndrome. The patient is normotensive and investigations show a hypochloraemic hypokalaemic alkalosis together with high urine potassium loss.

Bartter's syndrome is characterized by severe renal potassium wasting and an inability to concentrate the urine. Histologically, hyperplasia of the juxtaglomerular apparatus is seen.

The syndrome usually presents in childhood and an increased familial incidence has been noted. Children present with weakness, vomiting, polyuria, nocturnal enuresis, growth retardation and low IQ.

The diagnosis depends on demonstration of renal potassium loss in the presence of a hypokalaemic metabolic alkalosis, elevated aldosterone secretion and increased plasma renin activity, in a normotensive individual.

Abnormal potassium loss in the urine is suggested by the finding of more than 20 mmol of potassium in the urine per 24 hours with a plasma potassium of less than 3 mmol/l. Treatment consists of potassium supplementation with or without one aldosterone antagonist. Non-steroidal anti-inflammatory agents which interfere with tubular prostaglandin production have been shown to correct the hypokalaemic alkalosis and hyper-reninism. Some patients have hypomagnesaemia and require magnesium supplements.

The differential diagnosis of a metabolic hypokalaemic alkalosis includes:

1) Adrenal tumours^
2) Elevated ACTH levels
3) Diuretic abuse
4) Villous adenoma*
5) Laxative abuse*

^Blood pressure usually high
*Associated with diarrhoea and the urine potassium excretion is low.

13 a) The neuroleptic malignant syndrome is a well-recognized idiosyncratic side-effect of antidopaminergic drugs such as phenothiazines and butyrophenones which are used in the management of schizophrenia. The syndrome usually develops insidiously soon after treatment is initiated, and is characterized by hyperthermia, tachycardia, muscle rigidity, dysphagia and impaired consciousness. Creatinine kinase levels are elevated and reflect muscle damage. Death from respiratory failure is not uncommon; other complications include renal failure due to myoglobinuria, metabolic acidosis and cardiac failure. The increased muscle tone appears to be presynaptically mediated and recovery occurs when neuroleptic serum levels fall.

Management of the syndrome includes active cooling, rehydration and correction of metabolic acidosis, and ventilation when necessary. Intravenous dantrolene, which inhibits calcium efflux from muscle, and dopamine antagonists, e.g. bromocriptine, have been used with varying effect to reduce muscle tone.

14 a) A hypochloraemic hypokalaemic metabolic alkalosis.

b) Pyloric stenosis.

c) The patient's urine may be inappropriately acidic.

d) In pyloric stenosis, vomiting of HCl stomach contents occurs (no communication between stomach and duodenum) H^+ and Cl^- are lost and HCO_3^- is generated in the extracellular fluid resulting in a hypochloraemic alkalosis.

Urinary bicarbonate loss may be reduced in addition, due to: i) reduced GFR, and ii) a reduced chloride concentration in the glomerular filtrate, limiting resorption of sodium in the proximal tubule. More sodium is then available for exchange with H^+ and K^+, causing the urine to be inappropriately acid as H^+ secretion stimulates HCO_3^- reabsorption. The fall in chloride may also increase the loss of potassium in exchange for sodium.

As a result of these changes, there is a *rise* in plasma bicarbonate, a *rise* in pH, with a *fall* in chloride. A low potassium results from a combination of gut loss (though this will be less marked than in normal vomiting), alkalosis (resulting in loss into cells), and increased urinary loss as explained above.

15 a) De Quervain's thyroiditis (subacute thyroiditis). This occurs most commonly in young women. The exact aetiology is unknown, though a viral aetiology has been implicated. Often the initial presentation is of an upper respiratory tract infection with fever, sore throat and dysphagia. The thyroid gland is typically diffusely tender. Circulating thyroid hormone levels are high and signs of thyrotoxicosis may be present. Typically there is low or absent uptake of radioactive tracer on scanning.

b) The majority of cases respond to treatment with simple analgesics. Severe cases warrant a course of oral prednisolone. In the majority of cases the illness is short-lived and the patient is left euthyroid, but permanent hypothyroidism may result in some cases.

16 a i) Metastatic malignancy with widespread meningeal and base-of-skull deposits.
   ii) Motor Neurone Disease (MND).

b) Metastatic malignancy is the more likely — ptosis and upper cranial nerve signs are rare in MND.

c) Electromyography will facilitate the diagnosis of MND. Skull X-ray, CT brain scan and an isotope bone scan may be required to demonstrate meningeal or base-of-skull tumour deposits. Malignant cells may be found on CSF examination.

Motor neurone disease is a disease characterized by selective degeneration of the motor neurones involving both the corticospinal pathways and those originating in the motor nuclei of the brainstem and anterior horn cells of the spinal cord. The aetiology is uncertain apart from several rare familial varieties. Trauma, toxins and viruses may all be involved in susceptible individuals. It is slightly more common in men, symptoms usually arising between 50 and 70 years of age. The symptoms are usually insidious and depend on the relative predominance of lower and upper motor neurone symptoms. There are three main clinical pictures:

Progressive muscular atrophy
Progressive bulbar palsy
Amyotrophic lateral sclerosis.

The diagnosis is based on clinical findings of upper and lower motor neurone signs in the absence of sensory signs. Histologically the grey matter of the anterior horns is small and the anterior roots are wasted. In view of the inevitably fatal and progressive nature of the disease it is important that the diagnosis is established, and this is based on EMG findings of spontaneous fibrillation on mechanical stimulation, duration and amplitude of action potentials greater than normal and a marked reduction in the number of spikes on maximal contraction due to the decreased number of motor units available for contraction. The rate of progression of the condition is highly variable: progressive bulbar palsy has the worst prognosis (mean survival 2 years) and pure progressive muscular atrophy the best (survival up to 8 years).

17 a) The most likely diagnosis is coeliac disease — the symptoms were present long before his holiday in Malaysia. The history is entirely compatible with malabsorption. The proximal muscle weakness may be attributed to osteomalacia subsequent to vitamin D malabsorption — corrected serum calcium is low, serum phosphate is low and alkaline phosphatase is high.

b) i) The diagnosis of coeliac disease is confirmed by jejunal biopsy. The initial biopsy classically shows subtotal villous atrophy which subsequently improves on a gluten-free diet. In adults it is not necessary to re-biopsy after a trial reintroduction of gluten.

  ii) Measure serum levels of Vitamin B_{12}, folic acid, iron, TIBC and vitamin D.

c) The patient should be placed on a gluten-free diet. It may take up to 1 year for symptomatic improvement to occur. Dietary supplements of Vitamin D, folic acid and iron should be given; these become unnecessary once the patient has responded to the gluten-free diet.

  A differential diagnosis of the causes of subtotal villous atrophy includes:
1) Infectious enteritis in children
2) Giardiasis
3) Lymphoma
4) Whipple's disease
5) Hypogammaglobulinaemia
6) Cow's milk protein intolerance.

18 a) A is the interventricular septum. It is grossly thickened. Asymmetric septal hypertrophy is characteristic of hypertrophic obstructive cardiomyopathy. B is the closed mitral valve. The anterior movement of the mitral valve during systole is a feature of hypertrophic obstructive cardiomyopathy.

b) During systole, ventricular ejection occurs and must traverse the space between mitral valve apparatus and septum (space C). In hypertrophic obstructive cardiomyopathy this is narrowed and causes functional outflow obstruction. With squatting, the peripheral vascular resistance increases, and the corresponding increase in systolic blood pressure causes dilatation of the aortic root. This reduces the functional obstruction by increasing the space at C.

c) Atrial and ventricular arrhythmias are a feature of hypertrophic obstructive cardiomyopathy and usually underlie syncope. There is controversy as to whether functional outflow obstruction is ever significant enough to lead to syncope.

Answer to question 19

19 a) The most likely diagnosis is *Mycoplasma pneumoniae*.
The man presented with an atypical pneumonia associated with
hepatitis, erythema multiforme and cold agglutinins and
subsequently developed a myocarditis. Extrapulmonary
manifestations of *M. pneumoniae* occur in over 10% of cases,
generally within 3 weeks of the respiratory symptoms. The most
important complications in terms of morbidity and mortality are
cardiac (myocarditis and pericarditis) and neurological
(meningitis, meningo-encephalitis, ascending paralysis,
transverse myelitis, cranial nerve palsies, cerebellar ataxia and a
poliomyelitis-like illness). The other extrapulmonary problems
are more common, including skin rashes (25%), hepatitis,
pancreatitis (rare), cold agglutinins (50%), haemolytic anaemia,
bullous myringitis, thrombocytopenia, arthritis, and rarely,
glomerulonephritis.

b) i) To confirm a diagnosis of *M. pneumoniae*: isolation of the
organism from the respiratory system and mycoplasma
serology. Culture is slow and not always available. A
fourfold rise in antibody titre with a peak at 3–4 weeks
suggests a recent infection. A rise in the cold agglutinin
titre and the detection of specific IgM antibodies also suggest
recent infection.

ii) Tests to exclude other atypical infections including
legionnaire's disease, Q fever, psittacosis and viral
infections (Coxsackie A and B and CMV).

Treatment of *M. pneumoniae* is with erythromycin or
tetracycline. Early treatment probably decreases the frequency of
extrapulmonary complications, many of which are autoimmune
in origin.

20 a) Gilbert's syndrome. The only abnormality is an elevated
level of unconjugated bilirubin and the episode of jaundice was
preceded by loss of appetite and reduced calorie intake.

Gilbert's syndrome encompasses a number of inherited
metabolic abnormalities (presumed autosomal dominant in
nature) which result in mildly elevated levels of unconjugated
bilirubin. In many patients the primary defect is one of
conjugation due to low levels of bilirubin uridine diphosphate
glucoronate glucoronyl transferase. The elevated bilirubin level is
usually insufficient to produce clinical jaundice. The diagnosis is
usually made when calorie intake is reduced. This has the effect
of raising the serum levels of unconjugated bilirubin in the
absence of haemolysis. On reducing calorie intake to less than
400 calories, unconjugated bilirubin levels double in normal
patients and also those with Gilbert's disease. In the latter group,
due to the higher starting value, clinical jaundice is often
apparent.

A nicotinic acid provocation test may also be used to aid
diagnosis. Intravenous nicotinic acid elevates the level of
unconjugated bilirubin by at least 17 µmol/l and there is delayed
clearance compared to normal controls.

Liver biopsy is not essential for diagnosis; the histology is
usually unremarkable but may show an increase in centrilobular
lipofuscin. The long-term prognosis is excellent.

21 a) Rhabdomyolysis (with myoglobinuria)

b) Three possible reasons:
   i) status epilepticus
   ii) alcohol excess — note the low red cell transketolase level
      and elevated gamma glutamyl transpeptidase
   iii) a prolonged period of unconsciousness.

Rhabdomyolysis may also occur with sepsis, trauma, after
prolonged exertion and following burns and electrocution.
Biochemically it is characterized by a massively disproportionate
rise in serum creatinine from muscle damage compared with
blood urea, hyperkalaemia, increased muscle enzymes (AST and
CPK), hypocalcaemia as a consequence of calcium binding to
damaged muscle, and hyperuricaemia. Myoglobin is detected in
the urine and if in high enough concentration will turn the urine
red-brown. Myoglobinuria gives a false positive dipstick result for
blood but can be distinguished from haemoglobinuria by the
ammonium sulphate test, which gives a coloured precipitate with
haemoglobinuria and a coloured supernatant with
myoglobinuria. Treatment is principally supportive, although
alkalinization of the urine may ameliorate tubular damage and
the development of acute tubular necrosis; the renal lesion will
resolve spontaneously but a period of dialysis may be necessary.
Non-symptomatic hypocalcaemia should not be treated, as the
calcium will deposit uselessly in the muscle.

22 a) Lupus nephritis.

b) Sub-endothelial and intramembranous deposits typical of membranous glomerulonephritis.

c) The prognosis of nephritis in systemic lupus erythematosus is variable. Control of the patient's hypertension is important, and careful monitoring of renal function and protein excretion is necessary. Aggressive immunosuppressive therapy may be required.

There are three diseases in which linear IgG deposition may be reported on the glomerular basement membrane: i) anti-GBM disease (Goodpasture's syndrome), ii) diabetes mellitus, and iii) systemic lupus erythematosus. Goodpasture's syndrome is unlikely with this degree of hypertension and nephrotic range proteinuria, and diabetes mellitus is also unlikely with a normal glycosylated Hb level.

Lupus nephritis is now classified according to the histological features:

Class I — normal
Class IIa — electron microscopic or immunofluorescent evidence of mesangial disease
Class IIb — mesangial hypercellularity
Class III — focal segmental glomerulonephritis (<50% of glomeruli involved)
Class IV — diffuse glomerulonephritis (>50% of glomeruli involved)
Type V — membranous nephropathy.

Refractory hypertension is common in lupus nephritis and an important pitfall in its diagnosis is the apparently innocuous urinary sediment underlying an aggressive nephritis.

23 a) The glucose profile shows a lag storage pattern. The 30-minute sample is high and exceeds the renal threshold for glucose (usually 10 mmol/l) resulting in detectable glycosuria. This profile implies a delay in the hepatic storage of glucose. The initial high blood glucose levels lead to an increased insulin secretion which results in the subsequent hypoglycaemia.

b) The lag storage pattern may occur in apparently normal individuals but is a well-recognized complication of gastrectomy or gastrojejunostomy when rapid absorption of blood glucose occurs.

Other causes of a lag storage curve include severe liver disease associated with decreased glycogenolysis, and thyrotoxicosis.

Note: causes of a flat glucose tolerance curve where levels fail to rise normally following an oral glucose load include:

1) Normal individuals
2) Malabsorption states
3) Addison's disease
4) Hypopituitarism (with growth hormone deficiency).

24 a) This patient has had symptoms of malaise for 7 months, has several spider naevi and a biochemical hepatitis. The most likely diagnosis in this case is an **autoimmune chronic active hepatitis**. Vitiligo, the positive ANA and raised immunoglobulins all suggest an autoimmune aetiology.

The differential diagnosis of chronic hepatitis includes:
1) Autoimmune hepatitis (often associated with other autoimmune diseases)
2) Chronic viral hepatitis serological tests available for Hepatitis B, Hepatitis C and Hepatitis D.
3) Alcohol
4) Drugs, e.g. methyldopa, nitrofurantoin, and isoniazid
5) Wilson's disease
6) α_1 anti-trypsin deficiency.

Occasionally early primary biliary cirrhosis and primary sclerosing cholangitis may present with a biochemical hepatitis and be confused with chronic active hepatitis.

b) Appropriate investigations include a liver biopsy, organ-specific and non-organ-specific autoantibodies, anti-hepatitis C antibodies and serum caeruloplasmin and urinary copper estimation.

c) Immediate management would include stopping the contraceptive pill and alcohol, which may be contributing to the liver damage. Immunosuppression with corticosteroids forms the mainstay of treatment; azathioprine may be added as a steroid sparing agent.

Autoimmune chronic active hepatitis is commoner in women than in men and presents in two peaks, between 10 and 25 years of age and between 50 and 65 years of age. In addition to a biochemical hepatitis characterized by a raised aspartate amino-transferase level with a normal or only slightly elevated alkaline phosphatase, and the stigmata of chronic liver disease, 50% have other systemic symptoms including fever, arthralgia, vasculitic skin lesions, haemolytic anaemia, thrombocytopenia and leucopenia. A number of patients have other autoimmune diseases such as systemic lupus erythematosus, fibrosing alveolitis, diabetes mellitus, autoimmune thyroid disease, kerato-conjunctivitis sicca and ulcerative colitis. Typically patients have a positive ANA, raised immunoglobulins, primarily IgG, and a high titre of anti-smooth muscle antibodies. Recently antibodies against liver membrane and mitochondrial components (different from those found in primary biliary cirrhosis) have been detected, which appear to be specific for autoimmune chronic active hepatitis.

Liver histology shows inflammation in the portal and periportal areas with 'piecemeal' necrosis. In advanced disease liver architecture is disrupted and healing with fibrosis eventually leads to a macronodular cirrhosis.

25 a) The most likely diagnosis is **falciparum malaria** with acute tubular necrosis. The features suggesting malaria are:
1) An intermittent fever not responding to antibiotics, with a history of travel to a malaria region. The incubation period is normally 8–25 days; however, partial antimalaria prophylaxis and the non-specific features often result in considerable delay in presentation.
2) Frontal headaches, non-productive cough, myalgias and diffuse abdominal pains are typical of *Plasmodium falciparum*; chest pains and arthralgias are also recognized features. Malaria in the early stages may easily be confused with a viral illness.
3) Personality changes are the earliest signs of cerebral malaria. The lack of focal neurology, both on examination and on CT-scan, and the normal CSF findings make other diagnoses less likely.
4) The severity of the normochromic normocytic anaemia suggests malaria rather than another infection. Both haemolysis and dyserythropoiesis contribute to the anaemia in malaria. Massive haemolysis leads to haemoglobinuria, 'blackwater' fever.
5) Renal failure. Acute tubular necrosis is the main cause of acute renal failure in falciparum malaria. Several mechanisms contribute: i) intravascular haemolysis and haemoglobinuria, ii) hypovolaemia and renal vasoconstriction, and iii) blockage of small blood vessels. *Plasmodium malariae* and *Plasmodium falciparum* may cause a nephrotic syndrome, with evidence of immune complex deposition in the mesangium and glomerular basement membrane. A unique feature of falciparum malaria is that parasitized RBC have an increased ability to stick to endothelium; this is related to protuberances on the RBC surface expressing a molecule similar to thrombospondin which binds to fibronectin. Sequestration and blockage of parasitized RBC in capillaries of brain and kidney play an important role in damage to these organs.

b) Thick and thin blood films should be obtained to identify RBC parasites.
The differential diagnosis is obviously wide and includes other infections such as infective endocarditis and brucellosis. Syphilis, visceral Leishmaniasis, ascending cholangitis and AIDS are all very unlikely; the lack of lymph nodes or hepatosplenomegaly makes neoplasia (such as Hodgkin's disease) or sarcoidosis unlikely.

c) Treatment — cautious rehydration; intravenous quinine is given for 7 days followed by a single dose of pyrimethamine-sulfadoxine (Fansidar). Quinine levels should be measured to monitor therapy.

26 a) Digoxin, verapamil and adenosine cause AV nodal block and will increase the degree in this case or even cause complete AV dissociation.

Isoprenaline, atropine and imipramine will increase conduction through the node and might relieve the 2:1 block demonstrated.

27 a) Urinalysis and pregnancy test.

b) When was the patient's last menstrual period, and what contraception does she use?

c) This patient is pregnant. The alkaline phosphatase (ALP) is commonly moderately elevated due to placental production of this enzyme. Pregnancy is an anabolic state, and hepatic synthesis of many proteins (e.g. C3 and C4) is enhanced. However, the plasma volume is also increased, resulting in a dilutional anaemia and hypoalbuminaemia.

d) The commonest explanation for a low haemolytic complement level (CH50) with normal antigenic levels of individual components is in vitro complement activation. This occurs most frequently when blood samples take a long time to reach the laboratory, as occurred in this case. The low CH50 levels are thus an artefact of the collecting time.

Note: symptoms of carpal tunnel syndrome are common in pregnancy, and often respond to simple splinting.
Hyperpigmentation in a butterfly distribution is a well recognized complication of pregnancy.

28 a)   i)   **Anorexia nervosa** — the most common reason for weight loss in this age group.

      ii)   **Brucellosis** — she may have been drinking unpasteurized milk in Greece.

     iii)   **A second malignancy** — Hodgkin's disease is most likely with a history of fevers, and 10 years is an appropriate time interval.

   b)   i)   Admit for observation of eating pattern.

      ii)   Brucella antibody levels; IgG and IgM in acute infection, IgG and IgA in chronic infection.

The diagnosis of anorexia nervosa is a clinical one, based on the following findings: considerable weight loss, specific psychopathology associated with guilt about eating, loss of control and a disturbed body image where the patient perceives herself as fat. Patients diet excessively, excercise keenly and may have experienced a recent emotional upset. On examination the patient may have signs of extreme weight loss, blue-cold hands and feet, dry skin with downy hair over the nape of neck, cheeks, forearms and legs, and a low pulse pressure is often observed. LH, FSH and oestradiol levels are abnormally low. In the male, plasma LH and testosterone levels are low and there is loss of sexual interest and potency. Other blood results are likely to be normal unless self-induced vomiting is associated with electrolyte abnormalities. The increased incidence in Western society, and among higher social classes, suggest that the aetiology is related to culturally determined attitudes. The aims of treatment are to obtain the patient's confidence and a degree of cooperation, restore their weight to a healthy level, reduce residual disability and shorten the duration of the illness.

Brucellosis is a zoonosis caused by *Brucella melitensis, B. suis* or *B. abortus*, in decreasing order of frequency in man. The organism is a small Gram-negative coccobacillus which is an intracellular pathogen. Primary infection may be acute, chronic or subclinical. It may be contracted from milk or soft cheeses, tending animals and handling the carcasses of infected animals, and is an occupational disease of farmers and related professions. The bacillus enters across mucous membranes, is phagocytosed, reaches lymph nodes and there replicates. It is released when the cell is disrupted and reaches the liver and spleen.

Chills, sweats, aches and pains, general lethargy and episodic fevers are typical. Granulocytopenia may be the first clue to the diagnosis and lymphocytosis can occur when it is chronic. The diagnosis is made either serologically or by isolation of the organism from blood cultures, bone marrow aspirate, or pus.

Treatment is with tetracycline if the condition is diagnosed early, otherwise streptomycin must be added. Doxycycline and rifampicin are also an effective therapeutic combination. Spontaneous resolution occurs after months without treatment; relapse is common and may occur within 2 months of treatment.

29 a) The most likely diagnosis is Farmer's lung, an extrinsic allergic alveolitis, in which the patient is hypersensitive to spores of thermophyllic actiomycetes in mouldy hay. Extrinsic allergic alveolitis refers to a group of conditions in which inhaled organic dusts trigger a hypersensitivity reaction, including Farmer's lung, Bird-fancier's lung, Mushroom-worker's lung, etc. Although many of these conditions are associated with specific precipitins (antibodies to the presumed antigen), complement activation by immune complexes (type III hypersensitivity) is no longer thought to be the only or even the most important mechanism causing lung damage. Cell-mediated (type IV) hypersensitivity is probably the most important process. Histology shows extensive lymphocyte infiltration of the alveolar walls and in more advanced cases granuloma formation and lung fibrosis. The acute form presents as an influenza-like illness (malaise, myalgia, fever, headache) and breathlessness with a dry cough but no wheeze. The symptoms commence 3–9 hours after exposure to the sensitizing antigen. A period of exposure (several weeks to months) is required before the first attacks are noticed. In severe forms hypoxia may be profound and the chest X-ray shows a ground glass appearance. In the chronic form the symptoms are less dramatic and there is gradual onset of dyspnoea on exertion. The most consistent physical sign is fine crepitations heard throughout the lung. Patients may present with lung fibrosis or cor pulmonale which may be difficult to distinguish from cryptogenic fibrosing alveolitis or sarcoid. The fibrosis may be predominantly in the upper lobes and simulate the chest X-ray changes of tuberculosis.

b) The most important step is to take an occupational history to identify the causative antigen and confirm appropriate exposure. Further investigations should include a lung biopsy, bronchoalveolar lavage and examination of the serum for precipitating antibodies.

Investigation of extrinsic allergic alveolitis involves pulmonary assessment, antigen identification and history of relevant exposure, and finally immunological confirmation of the hypersensitivity. Lung function tests show a restrictive ventilatory defect with some air trapping and occasionally some evidence of large airways obstruction. Biopsy is the most sensitive way of distinguishing between cryptogenic fibrosing alveolitis, other granulomatous disease and extrinsic allergic alveolitis. Bronchoalveolar lavage findings are similar to sarcoid — with increased lymphocytes, unlike cryptogenic fibrosing alveolitis, where polymorphs predominate. The finding of precipitating IgG antibodies is not diagnostic since such antibodies are found in healthy people who have had appropriate exposure. If the diagnosis remains doubtful then challenge tests using inhaled antigen may be considered.

Treatment is avoidance of the responsible antigen. Steroids may be useful in a severe acute extrinsic allergic alveolitis. Patients are eligible for compensation under the Industrial Injuries Acts.

30 A

a) Autosomal dominant with inheritance.

B

a) From the family tree males are affected, and unaffected females are able to transmit the trait. Therefore the likely mode of transmission is X-linked recessive.

b) The risk to A and his children is zero as A will receive a Y chromosome from his affected father. We can assume the chance that a new mutation which would give rise to the same condition can be ignored. In the case of patient B, his great-grandfather was affected, implying that his grandmother was a carrier and therefore the probability that his mother was a carrier is 1/2; his risk is therefore 1/4. The mother of patient C has an affected brother, therefore the probability that she is a carrier is 1/2; the chance that her daughter will also be a carrier is 1/4.

c) The principal X-linked recessive conditions encountered are Haemophilia A and B, Duchenne and Becker's muscular dystrophy, glucose-6-dehydrogenase deficiency, nephrogenic diabetes insipidus, Hunter's syndrome, Lesch–Nyhan syndrome, colour blindness and Fabry's disease.

31 a) Post-infectious malabsorption syndrome (formerly called tropical sprue). Post-infectious malabsorption syndrome may be defined as a chronic malabsorption syndrome (greater than 2 months' duration) in which an abnormal bacterial flora — typically mixed aerobic enterobacteria — is present in the small intestine.

The disease is common in India, the Indian subcontinent, the West Indies and South America but less common in Africa, and occurs not only in travellers but also in the indigenous population.

The disease usually starts after several years' residence in the tropics, with an acute attack of diarrhoea believed to be infective in origin. This is followed by colonization of the small intestine with a mixed population of aerobic enterobacteria. Histologically there is evidence of mucosal damage, though villous atrophy is not a feature. Severe folic acid depletion is usually present by 4 months and exacerbates the mucosal damage. Plasma levels of enteroglucagon are high, which serves to reduce intestinal motility, encouraging the persistence of an abnormal flora.

Following the acute attack of diarrhoea which may be bloody, diarrhoea becomes chronic, with bulky stool, and colicky abdominal pain is common. Symptoms and signs are those of malabsorption and vitamin deficiencies. Fever, weight loss, pigmentation and glossitis are common. Folic acid deficiency is often severe and B_{12} deficiency may occur as in this case, resulting in dorsal column loss and loss of ankle jerks. Osteomalacia leads to proximal weakness.

The diagnosis may only be made when all other causes, especially infections with giardia and strongyloides, have been ruled out.

b) The differential diagnosis includes:
1) Coeliac disease
2) Crohn's disease
3) Infections:
   Giardia lamblia
   Strongyloides stercoralis
   Cryptosporidium
4) Small intestine lymphoma
5) Kwashiorkor
6) Ileocaecal tuberculosis
7) Hypolactasia.

c) Treatment regimen: a combination of tetracycline with folic acid supplementation usually results in rapid clinical improvement.

32 a) Lumbar spinal stenosis and claudication of the cauda equina.

b) Magnetic resonance imaging or myelography with or without CT-scanning are the investigations of choice. Surgery is the definitive treatment.

There are a number of mechanisms which may lead to stenosis of the lumbar canal, including osteoarthritis with hypertrophy of the facet joints, disc prolapse, surgery, spondylolisthesis, Paget's disease, neoplasia and infection. Any of these conditions may be superimposed on a congenitally narrow spinal canal.

Typically the symptoms develop slowly and may be very vague. Back pain as such is not a feature. The neurological symptoms often do not fit into any clear root or peripheral nerve distribution. In chronic cases there may be quadriceps wasting. The A–P diameter of the lumbar spinal canal is narrowed during extension, which appears to interfere with the blood supply to the cord; by stooping forward the A–P diameter is increased, so rapidly relieving the symptoms.

Normal plain radiographs of the spine do not exclude the diagnosis. Intermittent claudication may easily be distinguished from this syndrome by Doppler examination of the pulses before and after exercise.

33 a) End diastolic diameter exceeds 5.5 cm and there is therefore left ventricular dilatation.

b) Any space behind the posterior wall of the left ventricle is abnormal; it represents a pericardial effusion.

c) i) A paradoxical rise in the jugular venous pressure on inspiration — 'Kussmaul's sign'.

  ii) Pulsus paradoxus — an exaggerated fall in the systolic blood pressure on inspiration (normally less than 10 mmHg).

These signs only occur if there is significant haemodynamic compromise as a result of the effusion.

34 a) Gonococcal arthritis.

b) Investigations aim to isolate the organism (Gram-negative intracellular diplococci) from the urethra, vagina, throat, synovial fluid, blood, or from a pustule. Gonococci are notoriously difficult to grow in culture; blood cultures will be positive in less than 20% and synovial cultures in less than 50%.

Neisseria gonococci are a frequent cause of septic arthritis in young people. Radiology of the joint is normal unless the condition is left untreated, when severe destruction can take place.

Gonorrhoea occurs in females as frequently as in males; however, affected females generally have fewer symptoms and may act as asymptomatic carriers. Pregnant and menstruating females are more prone to haematogenous spread from vaginal foci. Arthritis and a vesiculopustular skin rash are the commonest complications. Others include endocarditis, meningitis, myocarditis, and hepatitis. A mild fever and leucocytosis, raised ESR and CRP accompany gonococcaemia. Tenosynovitis, particularly of the wrists, hands, feet or Achilles tendon, occurs in two-thirds of cases. Tenosynovitis, a fever and one or two swollen joints in a young person strongly suggest the diagnosis.

35 a) The clinical picture of an acute illness characterized by fever, a widespread rash, diarrhoea, myalgia, drowsiness and hypotension is typical of the **toxic shock syndrome**. The toxic shock syndrome, due to a toxin-producing staphylococcus, is usually associated with tampon use in menstruating females but can also occur in association with staphylococcal conjunctivitis, pharyngitis, infected burns and local abscesses.

Definitive criteria for the diagnosis include:
1) A temperature >39°C.
2) A widespread erythematous macular rash.
3) Hypotension systolic pressure <90 mmHg or a postural diastolic drop.
4) Toxic action on at least 3 systems, e.g. diarrhoea or vomiting, raised creatinine phosphokinase or myalgia, raised urea and creatinine, thrombocytopenia $<100 \times 10^9$/l, drowsiness and confusion.
5) A local source of infection — eyes, oropharynx, vagina, etc.

b) A vaginal examination should be performed and any tampon removed. The toxin-producing staphylococcus should be isolated from the primary site and/or the blood. Other infections such as streptococcal septicaemia, leptospirosis, measles and rickettsial infections must be excluded. A low threshold for examination of the cerebrospinal fluid should pertain if drowsiness is prominent.

c) Tampon removal prevents further absorption of toxin; parenteral flucloxacillin should be given initially and the specific sensitivity of the organism awaited. Shock should be treated with intravenous fluids and inotropic agents may be necessary.

36 A

a) Lithium toxicity would account for the drowsiness, tremor, thyroid function abnormalities and ECG changes.
Hypernatraemia complicates lithium-induced nephrogenic diabetes insipidus, when the patient's conscious level prevents an adequate fluid intake necessary to compensate for the polyuria.

Lithium is primarily used in the treatment of manic depressive illness. Lithium is excreted by the kidneys and has a low therapeutic index. Regular drug monitoring is recommended at monthly intervals.

Theraputic levels of lithium: 0.4–1.2 mmol/l. Toxicity occurs with levels >1.5 mmol/l and coma may occur with levels >2.5 mmol/l.

Recognized side-effects of lithium include fine tremor, nausea and diarrhoea, low T4 and compensatory rise in TSH. Hypothyroidism may be apparent; polyuria and polydypsia are common and a few patients develop frank diabetes insipidus (lithium antagonizes the effect of ADH on the distal convoluted tubule and collecting ducts). Lithium may also induce a state of partial renal tubular acidosis. Symptoms of lithium toxicity include drowsiness, coarse tremor, vomiting, coma, fits, renal failure and cardiovascular collapse.

Lithium toxicity may be provoked by sodium depletion. Eighty percent of lithium filtered by the glomerulus is reabsorbed by the proximal convoluted tubule and this percentage is increased in sodium-depleted states.

B

a) Hepatic encephalopathy due to alcoholic liver disease.

b) Hyponatraemia — secondary hyperaldosteronism.

Low urea — reduced hepatic synthesis.

Thrombocytopenia — hypersplenism.

Macrocytosis and increased triglyceride levels are commonly found in alcoholic patients.

37 a) The diagnosis is progressive systemic sclerosis.
Raynaud's phenomenon, pruritus, prolonged tanning and skin oedema are common features of early progressive systemic sclerosis. As the disease progresses major organs become involved, particularly the lungs, kidneys, gut and heart.

b) Complications:

1) Interstitial pneumonitis — she has shortness of breath on exertion, basal crackles and pulmonary function tests consistent with lung restriction (loss of lung volume and a reduced TLCO). Pulmonary manifestations, including interstitial pneumonitis, pulmonary fibrosis, pleural thickening and pleural effusions, are common in progressive systemic sclerosis and may occur early. Progressive interstitial lung disease may be complicated by pulmonary hypertension and right-sided heart failure, a frequent cause of death in progressive systemic sclerosis. Pulmonary hypertension secondary to an extensive pulmonary artery sclerosis may occur in the absence of pulmonary fibrosis. Treatment of interstitial pneumonitis and progressive lung fibrosis is immunosuppression with prednisolone and cytotoxic agents such as cyclophosphamide. A rare pulmonary complication of progressive systemic sclerosis is alveolar cell or bronchiolar carcinoma.

2) Renovascular hypertension — her blood pressure and her plasma creatinine levels are elevated (taking into consideration her age and urea level). Renovascular hypertension is generally a late but ominous complication of progressive systemic sclerosis, often leading to rapidly-progressive and irreversible renal failure. The onset of the hypertension is often sudden and may be heralded by headaches. Urgent control of the blood pressure as an inpatient is indicated. Often, even with control of the blood pressure, renal function continues to decline. Patients on corticosteroids appear to be more likely to present with malignant hypertension.

Answer to question 38

38 a) Hypogammaglobulinaemia with immunodeficiency. The clues are: chronic childhood infections (mostly bacterial), chronic diarrhoea which responds to antibiotics including metronidazole (*Giardia lamblia*), a chronic non-erosive arthritis and low immunoglobulins (normal albumin but a low total protein). An important differential diagnosis to consider is cystic fibrosis, but the low immunoglobulin level makes this unlikely.

b) Immunoglobulin levels, including subclasses.

c) Sandoglobulin (pooled human immunoglobulin) intravenously 2–4-weekly and penicillin V 500 mg daily.

The primary defect is unknown. Patients have normal numbers of B-cells and generally normal T-cell populations. There appears to be a defect in antibody production or secretion. Infections with pyogenic bacteria (particularly haemophilus, staphylococcus, streptococcus, and pseudomonas) and protozoa (*Giardia lamblia*) are the main clinical consequences of antibody deficiency. The majority of patients present in the second or third decade but any age is possible. (Note: they do not present before 3–6 months of age as maternal antibodies provide protection).

Lymphadenopathy is a common finding and typically histology shows granulomas.

Chronic respiratory tract infections may lead to bronchiectasis, pulmonary fibrosis, cor pulmonale and early death.

The polyarthritis/arthralgia associated with hypogammaglobulinaemia is a symmetrical non-erosive polyarthritis which generally spares the hands and feet. Tenosynovitis can be prominent; rarely, rheumatoid nodules are seen. Synovial histology shows a mononuclear cell infiltrate but not the lymphoid hyperplasia seen in rheumatoid arthritis. Rheumatoid factors are absent. It is always important to consider the possibility of septic arthritis (particularly mycoplasma) in these patients.

Chronic diarrhoea is a common feature and is often due to chronic giardia infection; similarly patients with selective IgA deficiency also have this complication.

B_{12} deficiency and atrophic gastritis occur, without the antibodies associated with pernicious anaemia.

There is an increased incidence of autoimmune disease and malignancy. The possibility of a lymphoma must be considered if lymphadenopathy is a major feature. B_{12} deficiency and atrophic gastritis are not uncommonly seen in these patients.

39 a) Disseminated intravascular coagulation complicating acute promyelocytic leukaemia. The coagulation tests are diagnostic of disseminated intravascular coagulation, a well-recognized complication of acute promyelocytic leukaemia.

The characteristic coagulation abnormalities are thrombocytopenia (this may also be caused by infiltration of the marrow with blasts), prolongation of the prothrombin, partial thromboplastin and thrombin times, hypofibrinogenaemia and raised levels of fibrin degradation products.

b) The diagnosis of acute myeloid leukaemia can be confirmed by bone marrow examination which will reveal the characteristic hypergranular blasts. The granules contain a procoagulant which triggers disseminated intravascular coagulation, which may be the presenting feature of this type of leukaemia. Lysis of the blasts during chemotherapy may worsen the disseminated intravascular coagulation and treatment must include meticulous monitoring of coagulation and appropriate support with platelets and fresh frozen plasma. The role of heparin is controversial. Once in remission, acute promyelocytic leukaemia has one of the most favourable prognoses of AML.

Recognized causes of acute disseminated intravascular coagulation include:

1) *Infections and toxins*
   Gram-negative septicaemia, malaria, snake bite
2) *Malignancy*
   Disseminated malignancy, acute promyelocytic leukaemia
3) *Obstetric causes*
   Amniotic fluid embolism, abruptio placentae, retained fetus, eclampsia, antepartum haemorrhage
4) *Miscellaneous*
   Mismatched transfusion, major trauma, aortic dissection.

40 A
a) Measurement of lung volumes TLC/RV to assess hyperinflation and air trapping.
Bronchodilator response.

b) Emphysema.

B
a) Right pneumonectomy.

C a) Ventilatory failure.

b) Compensated respiratory acidosis.

41 a) Pyrexia; neck stiffness; focal neurological deficit; signs of ear or upper respiratory tract infection; papilloedema.

b) FBC, blood cultures, biochemical profile, blood glucose, head CT scan, lumbar puncture and CSF examination. There may be organisms visible on a Gram stain of the CSF, and neutrophils in the CSF, with a raised protein and low sugar. These findings indicate bacterial meningitis. A lymphocytosis suggests TB or more commonly, viral meningitis. Chemotherapy would be modified in the light of the microscopy and later culture results. The probable diagnosis is **meningococcal meningitis**.

c) Therapy with broad spectrum antibiotics, usually intravenous benzyl penicillin and chloramphenicol (or new generation cephalosporins). Some neurological centres also recommend starting acyclovir, particularly if there was any delay in obtaining the CSF results. Death; fits; residual neurological deficit; deafness; hydrocephalus; DIC; digital gangrene following vascular occlusion; circulatory collapse; Waterhouse–Friedrichsen syndrome; renal failure.

d) Immunoglobulins and serum complement estimation. Terminal pathway (C5–C8) complement deficiency predisposes particularly to meningococcal infection.

Typical CSF findings

	Pressure	Leucocytes	Protein	Glucose
Viral meningitis	Normal/ mild increase	50–500/mm lymphocytes	0.4–1 g/l	normal
Note: PMN may be increased during the first 24–48 hours. CSF glucose levels may be low in cases of mumps or herpes meningitis.				
Bacterial meningitis	Elevated	500–2000/mm³ PMN	1–5 g/l	Very low
Tuberculous meningitis	Elevated	50–500/mm³ lymphocytes	1–5 g/l	Usually low
Note: PMN may be increased during the first 24–48 hours.				
Cryptococcal meningitis	Elevated	5–500/mm³ lymphocytes	0.5–5 g/l	Usually low
Carcinomatous meningitis (malignant cells often found)	N/elevated	5–300/mm³ lymphocytes	0.5–5 g/l	Normal/ reduced

42 a) Sexual history — he has just been to Bangkok; a history of urethritis.

b) Reiter's syndrome. Gonococcal infection.

c) The classic Reiter's triad consists of arthritis, conjunctivitis and urethritis. The seronegative arthritis typically affects the large and small joints of the lower limbs in an asymmetrical fashion; sacroileitis is common. Conjunctivitis and urethritis are usually mild.

Other recognized clinical features include plantar fasciitis, Achilles tendonitis, keratoderma blenorrhagica, circinate balanitis and painless buccal ulcers.

The initial disease is usually self-limiting but the arthritis becomes chronic in up to 60% of cases. Other late manifestations include uveitis, aortic regurgitation, conduction defects, pericarditis, pulmonary infiltrates, peripheral neuropathy and central nervous system involvement.

d) i) HLA-B27. Between 70 and 90% of patients with Reiter's syndrome are HLA-B27 positive.

ii) Attacks may occur following intestinal infections, e.g. *Shigella flexneri* and *dysenteriae* (not *sonnei*), salmonella, yersinia and campylobacter.

43 a) The presence of polycythaemia with splenomegaly is highly suggestive of **primary proliferative polycythaemia** (polycythaemia rubra vera) a myeloproliferative disorder caused by the autonomous proliferation of a clone of erythroid cells which occurs in the absence of any erythropoietin drive. The diagnosis is supported by the elevated white cell and platelet counts and the raised serum urate (though in this case the patient's elevated uric acid level could be due to the thiazide diuretics or alcohol). There is no evidence of dehydration and blood gases are normal.

Polycythaemia refers to an increase in the haemoglobin concentration:

	Males	**Females**
Hb	>17.5 g/dl	>15.5 g/dl
Red cell count	>6 × 10^{12}/l	>5.5 × 10^{12}/l
Haematocrit	>55%	>47%

Causes of polycythaemia may be subdivided into:
1) **Primary proliferative polycythaemia**
2) **Secondary causes**
    i) Inappropriate erythropoietin production, e.g. renal cysts, hypernephroma, cerebellar haemangioblastoma, hepatocellular carcinoma, uterine fibromas
    ii) Compensatory increased erythropoietin production, e.g. high altitude, alveolar hypoventilation, cyanotic heart disease, smoking, methaemoglobinaemia.
3) **Relative polycythaemia**
    Due to reduced plasma volume, e.g. dehydration, diuretics.

b) The first aim in the investigation of polycythaemia is to distinguish the condition caused by a true increase in red cell mass from relative polycythaemia, caused by a contraction of the plasma volume rather than any true increase in red cell mass. This may be achieved by isotopic measurement of red cell mass and plasma volume. Having established absolute polycythaemia, primary polycythaemia needs to be distinguished from the secondary causes.

Further appropriate investigations include:
1) Bone marrow examination — hypercellular with prominent megakaryocytes in primary proliferative polycythaemia — and detection of erythropoietin-independent bone forming units.
2) Serum vitamin B_{12} binding capacity is high in primary proliferative polycythaemia.
3) Serum erythropoietin levels are normal or low in primary proliferative polycythaemia and high in other cases of secondary polycythaemia. In some patients further investigations to determine the source of inappropriately high erythropoietin levels will be necessary.

Treatment options for primary proliferative polycythaemia include venesection, cytotoxic drugs, e.g. chlorambucil and busulphan, and Phosphorus-32 therapy.

44 There is pulmonary hypertension with a right-to-left shunt. The most common cause is an **Eisenmenger ventricular septal defect.**

a) A right atrial pressure as high as this almost certainly suggests tricuspid regurgitation, secondary to right ventricular dilation and dysfunction. The waveform would be a dominant systolic wave, which is variously described as a V-wave, S-wave or delta wave.

b) The low pulmonary artery diastolic pressure suggests pulmonary regurgitation. This often occurs as a result of prolonged pulmonary hypertension. There is no systolic gradient.

c) At 1 year the shunt would be left to right, and the pulmonary arterial tree is more prominent than usual in these circumstances ('pulmonary plethora'). With the onset of pulmonary hypertension of suprasystemic levels, blood is diverted from right to left and away from the lungs giving oligaemia ('peripheral pruning') and the hilar pulmonary artery shadows become greatly enlarged.

Note: closure of the ventricular septal defect at this stage would lead to rapid death from right ventricular failure. With pulmonary vascular resistance of this magnitude the right ventricle is protected from fatal dilation and failure by the 'offloading' effect of the tricuspid incompetence and the systolic right-to-left shunt.

45 a) The patient's fluid balance charts should be studied carefully. The precise anti-TB drugs he has been taking, and the duration of therapy, should be ascertained.

b) Acute interstitial nephritis — Rifampicin is a likely cause. A hypersensitivity aetiology is thought likely and this is supported by the frequent association of fever, arthralgia, rash, peripheral eosinophilia and eosinophiluria. Oliguria, salt and potassium loss due to tubular dysfunction and modest proteinuria are typical features. Some patients may be polyuric.

c) Full serum biochemical profile, including sodium, calcium, phosphate, and liver function test; full blood count — an eosinophilia is typical.

d) Renal ultrasound and biopsy. Renal biopsy typically shows a cellular infiltrate composed primarily of eosinophils, with superadded tubular necrosis. In some patients linear deposition of IgG and C3 along the tubular basement membrane has been shown.

e) Modification of the anti-TB treatment regime. Corticosteroids, e.g. Prednisolone 60 mg/day, may lead to more rapid recovery of renal function. Correction of electrolyte imbalance is necessary and acute renal replacement therapy may be required. In most patients full recovery of renal function occurs.

Previous peritoneal TB is a contraindication to acute peritoneal dialysis, and haemodialysis would need to be performed on a unit accepting HBsAg-positive patients.

Answer to questions 46–47

46 a) Non-sustained ventricular tachycardia.
   b) None. The treatment of non-sustained ventricular tachycardia has not been shown to improve prognosis in heart failure.

47 a) The patient is describing **two transient ischaemic attacks** involving the **carotid territory**. The visual symptoms are usually described as *amaurosis fugax*. The short duration, and nature of onset, are typical — description of a blind or curtain coming across the field of vision is classical.

   b) Has he experienced other attacks in the carotid territory, or in other vascular territories, e.g. vertebrobasilar, characterized by hemisensory disturbance or hemiparesis, diplopia, dizziness, nausea, ataxia, or dysarthria? Is there a relevant family history of stroke, or cardiac disease? Is there a history of smoking, hypertension, diabetes, angina, blackouts, claudication, or other systemic disease associated with arteritis? Were there any specific events that precipitated the attacks; any history of chest pain or palpitations, headache, sudden movement or anything to precipitate a fall in blood pressure (e.g. anti-hypertensive drugs)?

   c) Lying and standing BP in both arms should be measured; bruits should be sought in all vascular territories; full cardiac examination, to exclude valvular pathology — about 30% of TIA patients have a potential cardiac source of embolism; splinter haemorrhages, other signs of endocarditis or evidence of a systemic vasculitis may sometimes be found; residual abnormal neurological signs are not generally found, but careful fundoscopy is required — platelet or cholesterol emboli may be present in the retinal arterioles.

   d) The cause of the TIA should be sought — history and examination, as above, will often provide useful pointers. Relevant investigations are FBC, ESR, biochemical profile, blood glucose, fasting lipids, VDRL, urinalysis, CXR, ECG and CT scan. Echocardiography or 24-hour ECG monitoring may be appropriate. Digital subtraction angiography of the great vessels is appropriate in a young patient with suspected carotid disease, in whom surgery is being considered.
   Medical treatment comprises: i) control of risk factors: BP, diabetes, hyperlipidaemia, obesity, smoking; ii) anti-platelet therapy with aspirin; iii) appropriate therapy for cardiac arrhythmias, or valve disease if relevant.

   e) Myocardial infarction.

48 a) The combination of thrombocytopenia, renal failure and cholestatic jaundice in a trout farmer is highly suggestive of **leptospirosis (Weil's disease)**. It is unusual for the other causes of jaundice such as viral hepatitis, infectious mononucleosis, malaria, Legionnaire's disease or brucellosis to present with this triad but these diagnoses should be actively excluded. Leptospirosis, a spirochaetal disease (caused by the *Leptospira interrogans* complex) is carried by rodents and usually passed to humans by contact with rat urine or blood, typically occurring in those exposed to rat excreta in the context of their occupation.

The clinical presentation varies from the classic picture of Weil's disease with multi-organ involvement, to a mild anicteric febrile illness. Clinical features include fever, lymphadenopathy, headache, photophobia, conjunctival injection, abdominal pain, splenomegaly and profound myalgia. Renal involvement occurs in approximately 50% of cases and varies from mild proteinuria to dialysis-dependent renal failure. Jaundice occurs in 10% of cases and is typically cholestatic. Pulmonary involvement is common, though the severity varies from a dry cough to marked pulmonary infiltration with respiratory failure.

b) The diagnosis of leptospirosis may be made in the first 10 days of the illness by culture of blood or cerebrospinal fluid. Urine cultures become positive from the 2nd week. Serological diagnosis is possible after the 10th day using a macroscopic slide agglutination test or rising antibody titres. A peripheral blood polymorphonuclear leucocytosis is usual.

The cerebrospinal fluid findings — a normal sugar, slightly elevated protein with a lymphocyte pleocytosis, though initially neutrophils may predominate.

c) Penicillin or tetracyclines should be given within the first 5 days of the illness. Supportive treatment with attention to fluid balance is essential. Dialysis may be necessary. Overall the prognosis is good; poor prognostic factors include severe jaundice, disseminated intravascular coagulation, renal failure and respiratory failure.

49 a) Rupture of the oesophagus. The occurrence of severe retrosternal chest pain in a hypertensive smoker is obviously suggestive of myocardial ischaemia. However, the radiation of cardiac pain to the back is unusual in an uncomplicated myocardial infarction and is more compatible with aortic dissection. Against the diagnosis of aortic dissection is the lack of pulse inequality, the absence of aortic incompetence and the presence of a left pleural effusion.

The history of pain starting during a meal, and radiating through to the back coupled with the presence of a left pleural effusion in a shocked patient, is highly suggestive of a ruptured oesophagus.

b) The diagnosis may be confirmed by gastrograffin examination of the oesophagus, which will demonstrate the presence of a tear.

50 a) Phenytoin toxicity presenting with cerebellar syndrome, mild megaloblastic anaemia and osteomalacia. The recent fit might be paradoxical, i.e. related to high phenytoin levels. Rifampicin is an enzyme inducer and unlikely to be responsible for high phenytoin levels unless the dosage of phenytoin had been increased to compensate.

b) Investigations should include measurement of plasma phenytoin level, serum folate and vitamin B_{12} and vitamin D levels.

The principal side-effects of phenytoin include:

1) Central nervous system — cerebellar signs, typically ataxia, tremor, nystagmus and dysarthria; sedation; mood swings; peripheral neuropathy; increased fits
2) Haematological — folate deficiency leading to a megaloblastic anaemia; aplastic anaemia; lymphadenopathy
3) Endocrine — increased metabolism of vitamin D which may lead to osteomalacia; reduced ADH levels, worsening of diabetes mellitus
4) Skin — acne; coarsening of facial features; gum hypertrophy; Dupuytren's contractures
5) Hepatitis
6) Drug-induced LE
7) Drug fever
8) Fetal abnormalities — microcephaly, congenital heart disease, cleft palate and hare lip.

There is a large genetic variation in the rate of phenytoin metabolism, so that monitoring levels is essential. A number of drugs impair phenytoin metabolism, including isoniazid, chloramphenicol, and dicoumarol. Ethanol and carbamazepine increase phenytoin metabolism.

Note: Phenytoin is an enzyme inducer and will increase the metabolism of drugs such as the oral contraceptive pill.

51 A
a) **Pulmonary vascular disease**, e.g. multiple pulmonary emboli Primary pulmonary hypertension Right-to-left shunt
b) Echocardiogram; cardiac catheter.

B
a) **Pulmonary fibrosis** secondary to rheumatoid arthritis.
b) CT scan, bronchoalveolar lavage, open lung biopsy.

52 a) Diplopia, aggressive/uninhibited behaviour, nystagmus, confusion, slurred speech, dehydration.

b) A history or signs of a head injury, e.g. skull fracture, subdural or extradural haemorrhage or other injury should be sought. Consider the possibility of ingestion of other drugs — e.g. barbiturates, heroin, antihistamines, methanol, ethylene glycol, cocaine, 'crack'. Look at the pupils, look for needle marks, talk to the police or to friends who may accompany the patient; consider hypoglycaemia or other metabolic upset.

c) Hypoglycaemia; rhabdomyolysis; fits; inhalation; peptic ulceration; pancreatitis; irreversible brain damage; liver failure; hallucinations/tremor; Wernicke's encephalopathy; and Korsakoff's psychosis.

d) Ensure that the patient's airway remains patent; keep him hydrated; be aware of the risks of hypoglycaemia; treat fits and withdrawal symptoms as required; Vitamin B replacement (primarily thiamine). Consider appropriate psychiatric assessment or specialist counselling if the problem is one of chronic alcohol abuse.

53 a) Benign intracranial hypertension. The syndrome of an elevation in CSF pressure in the absence of ventricular dilation or intracerebral mass.

Benign intracranial hypertension is predominantly a disease of obese females. The aetiology is unknown, though associations with pregnancy, drugs (e.g. tetracyclines, nalidixic acid), dural sinus thrombosis, previous head injury and vitamin A deficiency states have been noted. Neurological signs are usually confined to swollen discs, though a partial VI nerve palsy is often found. A space-occupying lesion must be excluded.

b) CT scan — the ventricles will not be displaced, and may be normal or small. The diagnosis is confirmed by finding an elevated cerebrospinal fluid pressure. Dural sinus thrombosis should be excluded by angiography.

c) Visual loss due to optic atrophy. Permanent visual loss occurs in up to 50% of cases and may be severe in 10%.

d) Weight loss and diuretics form the mainstay of treatment. First, therapeutic lumbar punctures may be performed and high-dose corticosteroids have been used initially to reduce intracranial pressure effectively. Surgery is not usually required, though ventriculoperitoneal shunting of cerebrospinal fluid may be needed if visual loss is progressive and the response to steroids is slow.

Most cases undergo clinical remission either spontaneously or in response to treatment, though CSF pressure may remain high.

54 a) In the presence of acute chest pain the anterior changes are likely to represent left anterior descending (LAD) coronary artery occlusion. There is an inferior infarct of indeterminate age which probably results from right coronary artery occlusion.

b) The appearance of Q-waves early in an infarction is one feature of thrombolysis.

c) The atrioventricular node is an inferior structure. Its involvement in an anterior myocardial infarction is evidence of an extensive area of damage and is a poor prognostic sign.

d) Persistent ST segment elevation at 1 year strongly suggests the presence of a left ventricular aneurysm.

55 a) Intracardiac right-to-left shunting. The most marked effect of a shunt on saturation is in the chamber beyond that receiving the shunted blood; in this case that is the femoral artery, suggesting a ventricular septal defect.

b) There is a marked peak-to-peak systolic gradient across the pulmonary valve, indicating stenosis.

c) Overriding aorta. There is demonstrable ventricular septal defect, pulmonary stenosis and right ventricular hypertrophy; the most likely diagnosis is Fallot's tetralogy.

d) Dizzy spells may represent:
1) Increased right-to-left shunting with reduced peripheral vascular resistance (exercise) and therefore increasing systemic desaturation.
2) Recurrent paradoxical emboli are common due to polycythaemia and the right-to-left shunt.
3) Recurrent paroxysmal arrhythmias as a result of atrial distension.

56 a) Multiple sclerosis — retrobulbar neuritis.

b) Diminished acuity and colour vision in the affected eye, particularly centrally. Peripheral vision may be retained; the optic disc may be swollen. Examination of both eyes may reveal nystagmus and/or an internuclear ophthalmoplegia.

c) The episode of 'foot dragging' is explicable by the presence of a spinal cord plaque. Brainstem involvement often produces symptoms which may be confused with vestibular neuronitis. Such a relapsing/remitting course is typical of demyelinating disease.

d) Visual evoked responses; auditory evoked responses; CSF examination for evidence of local IgG synthesis; NMR scanning if available.

e) Acuity may return to normal over a few months, though there may be residual impairment of colour vision; recurrent attacks can occur. The temporal half of the optic disc (containing macular fibres) will be pale.

57 a) Hypocalcaemia due to hypoparathyroidism. The biochemical findings of hypocalcaemia with an elevated phosphate and a normal alkaline phosphatase (normal for an 8-year-old) are typical.

b) The differential diagnosis includes primary hypoparathyroidism and pseudohypoparathyroidism (the typical phenotype of pseudohypoparathyroidism includes an oval face and short 4th and 5th metacarpal bones).

These may be differentiated by:

1) Measurement of serum PTH levels — absent in primary hypoparathyroidism, and present in pseudohypo-parathyroidism, where the abnormality is a failure to respond to PTH.

2) The diagnosis of pseudohypoparathyroidism may be confirmed by the Ellsworth Howard test — a PTH infusion fails to increase urine phosphate and cyclic AMP, in contrast to primary hypoparathyroidism where both are elevated.

58 a) There is a significant gradient between the left atrial pressure (pulmonary capillary wedge) and left ventricle at end-diastole, indicating **mitral stenosis.**

b) The A-wave is a measurement of pressure at peak atrial contraction. The most common cause of an exaggerated A-wave is a hypertrophied and thus poorly compliant ventricle. In this case the right ventricle is clearly hypertrophied in response to pulmonary arterial hypertension.

c) Three features of palpation:

1) A palpable impulse of mitral valve closure (first heart sound) — 'tapping apex'.

2) A left parasternal systolic heave (right ventricular hypertrophy).

3) A palpable impulse of pulmonary valve closure (second heart sound) at high left parasternal area, a consequence of pulmonary hypertension.

d) A-waves only occur with atrial contraction — therefore sinus rhythm.

59 a) The differential diagnosis is of a single pulmonary nodule associated with linear shadowing, and a granulomatous reaction. The most likely diagnosis in this case is chronic infection caused by **histoplasmosis.**

Histoplasma capsulatum may cause an acute pneumonia or chronic pulmonary lesions. In endemic areas (such as Southern USA) the majority of those exposed never develop overt signs of infection unless they become immunosuppressed. Bird and bat excreta may contain large numbers of the organisms, and a history of inhalation of dust from a cave containing bats (as in this case), or a bird-house, is often noted in acute histoplasmosis. The acute illness occurs 2–3 weeks after exposure. The radiological changes tend to be out of proportion to the relatively mild symptoms. Cultures are typically negative. A rising complement fixation titre confirms the diagnosis. The pneumonia often settles without treatment and when acute is unresponsive to conventional antibiotics. In severe cases intravenous amphotericin B is given. Acute re-infection may cause acute bilateral pulmonary infiltrates and breathlessness. Chronic pulmonary disease is unusual but is recognized especially in male smokers. Progressive disease requires amphotericin B. Coin lesions may cavitate, or more commonly calcify. Rarely, patients may present with mediastinitis and SVC obstruction, or disseminated disease.

b) The other possibilities include:
1) Malignancy: a primary carcinoma or a metastasis (colon, kidney, germ-cell, melanoma, prostate or bone are the most likely in a man of this age).
2) A hypersensitivity reaction and fibrosis related to dust inhalation. However, typically both lungs would be affected.
3) Wegener's granulomatosis restricted to the lungs may occur but is extremely rare.
4) A chronic infection with acid-fast bacilli is unlikely since the organism has not been detected and the tuberculin test is negative.
5) Sarcoidosis — this would be a very atypical presentation of sarcoidosis.

c) Further investigations should include: i) complement fixation tests for fungi, particularly histoplasmosis and coccidioidomycosis; ii) culture of the biopsy material for fungi; the organisms may be difficult to detect even with specific stains in fibrosed material; iii) a thoracotomy and biopsy of the nodule to exclude malignancy and obtain material in which the yeasts should be easily seen using appropriate stains.

60 a) Osteonecrosis (avascular necrosis) of the femoral head.
Head of the humerus, medial and lateral condyles of the distal
femur, superior margin of the talus may also be affected.
b) Plain X-rays of both hips. The plain X-ray is often initially
normal but may show an infarcted area with surrounding
radiolucency, a sclerotic rim around the lesion, loose fragments
of bone, or fractures.

An isotope bone scan is the test of choice and will initially
show an area of reduced uptake which may be surrounded by
increased tracer localization. As repair gets under way, or if there
is extensive damage (with a fracture, for example) there may be
generally increased uptake.

c) The patient received an excess of steroid. A more usual
regimen would be hydrocortisone 20 mg in the morning, 10 mg
at night. High dose steroids are the most important cause of
osteonecrosis, and in this patient may have contributed both
directly and indirectly by causing weight gain.

Factors implicated in the pathogenesis of osteonecrosis
include:

1) Trauma, e.g. fracture — called avascular necrosis
2) Excess corticosteroids
3) Sickle cell disease
4) Deep sea diving
5) Radiotherapy
6) Alcohol
7) Pregnancy
8) Rheumatic diseases, e.g. rheumatoid arthritis,
    systemic lupus erythematosus
9) Hereditary disorders, e.g. Fabry's disease, Gaucher's
    disease, hyperlipidaemia
10) Infection, e.g. infective endocarditis.

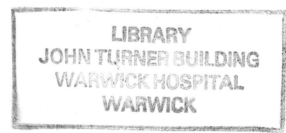

61 A

a) Acute pancreatitis. The low albumin, low corrected calcium, hypoxia and high blood glucose all point to the diagnosis, which may be confirmed by measurement of serum amylase levels; a level >1000 Somogyi units is said to be diagnostic.

b) Thiazide diuretics are a recognized cause of acute pancreatitis. Other drugs which may precipitate an acute attack include steroids, azathioprine and the contraceptive pill. In the UK the majority of cases of acute pancreatitis are idiopathic — the commonest-known precipitating cause is gallstones; other precipitating factors include alcohol, viral infections particularly mumps, trauma — which may be local, e.g. following ERCP or following general surgery — carcinoma of the pancreas, hyperparathyroidism and hypertriglyceridaemia.

B

a) Intracranial tumour, localized probably to the frontal cortex.

b) A fit *de novo* in a patient of this age always raises the suspicion of a space-occupying lesion. A previous history of headaches is important. Intellectual impairment, mood change, particularly euphoric or impulsive behaviour, are all typical of frontal lobe lesions.

c) Most intracranial tumours are secondary; FBC, ESR, full biochemical screen, and chest X-ray should be performed, together with a CT brain scan.

62 a) Thyroid crisis or thyroid storm. There is a family history of autoimmune disease and a good history of progressive weight loss — an indication of hyperthyroidism. The acute deterioration followed an upper respiratory tract infection and the patient presented with the classic combination of i) fever;
ii) cardiovascular symptoms — arrhythmias and hypotension;
iii) neurological involvement — confusion, agitation; and
iv) gastrointestinal involvement with abdominal pain and vomiting.

b) The condition is a medical emergency.
Management steps: Intravenous β-blockers — propranolol 2 mg i.v. is effective in relieving fever and tachycardia. 20 mg of carbimazole by nasogastric tube, repeated 4-hourly, or an equivalent dosage of propylthiouracil.

In some centres sodium iodide is given 1 hour after the first dose of carbimazole to prevent further release of thyroid hormones.

General supportive treatment; intravenous fluids; the patient may need appropriate sedation and digoxin may be necessary to control the atrial fibrillation.

Blood should be sent for measurement of thyroid hormones and thyroid autoantibodies.

63 a) Blood tests: Clotting screen, antiphospholipid antibodies, and lupus anticoagulant.
Radiological: Duplex doppler of the leg vessels, and a venogram should be considered.

b) Deep venous thrombosis in association with primary antiphospholipid syndrome. Differential diagnosis is Baker's cyst. The patient is a keen athlete and this occurs in traumatic and degenerative disease of the knee. The patient's positive VDRL may be related to treponemal infection, but a false positive VDRL occurs in patients with antiphospholipid antibodies and lupus-like illnesses.

c) If the diagnosis of a deep venous thrombosis is confirmed, the following should be done: full clotting screen with measurement of antithrombin III, protein S and C, and Factor V_{Leiden} should be undertaken. Measurement of antibodies to extractable nuclear antigens, complement levels, and DNA binding are also indicated, and a haemoglobin electrophoresis is required. He needs to have specific syphilis serology. It should not be forgotten that thromboses may occur in association with malignant disease, particularly adenocarcinomas.

d) If a diagnosis of primary antiphospholipid syndrome is confirmed he should be anticoagulated for life, maintaining an INR of 2.5–3.5. Follow-up in a specialist clinic is advisable.

64 A

a) The combination of acute abdominal pain, vomiting, epilepsy and a predominant motor neuropathy suggest the diagnosis of **acute intermittent porphyria**. This diagnosis is further supported by the hyponatraemia, raised serum bilirubin and aspartate trans-aminase levels.

b) Measure i) urine-δ-aminolaevulinic acid, and ii) urinary porphobilinogen. Both should be greatly raised during the acute attack; levels are also raised during remission. The addition of Ehrlich's aldehyde reagent to the urine should result in a pink colour due to the presence of porphobilinogen. A similar result is also obtained if the urine contains urobilinogen. The addition of n-butanol distinguishes porphobilinogen, which is insoluble in n-butanol, unlike urobilinogen which is soluble.

B

a) Galactosaemia (an autosomal recessive disorder): incidence 1:60 000 due to deficiency of the enzyme galactose-1-phosphate uridyl transferase. Deficiency of this enzyme results in high levels of galactose-1-phosphate which is thought to be responsible for organ damage.

b) Clinical features manifest soon after birth and include failure to thrive, vomiting, diarrhoea, hepatomegaly, jaundice, hypoglycaemia, cataracts, a Fanconi-type syndrome and psychomotor retardation. A well-recognized late complication, especially in girls, is hypergonadotrophic hypogonadism.

c) The diagnosis should be confirmed by measuring erythrocyte enzyme levels of galactose-1-phosphate uridyl transferase activity. Blood and urine galactose levels are raised in this condition.

d) Galactose should be excluded from the diet, probably for life. In infancy a milk substitute such as Nutramigen may be used. Treatment should be monitored by measuring erythrocyte levels of galactose-1-phosphate.

65 a) The patient has a progressive neurological disorder involving the brainstem (by vertigo and tinnitus) and cerebellum (dysarthria, ataxia and nystagmus). She also has weight loss, ascites and a cystic lesion affecting the right ovary. CT scan shows cortical and cerebellar atrophy. The most likely diagnosis is a **paraneoplastic syndrome involving the cerebellum and brainstem**, associated with an **ovarian neoplasm**. Carcinoma of the bronchus is also a possibility but this patient was a non-smoker and the chest X-ray is normal apart from old tuberculous apical changes

The CSF protein and cell count is raised, so the differential diagnosis should include chronic meningitis due to fungus, tuberculosis or carcinoma. However, such diseases typically cause cranial nerve palsies or focal problems due to infiltration or a mass effect. Lymphomas cause meningeal infiltration and are also associated with more frequent opportunistic infections of the central nervous system (Listeria, cryptoccocus, toxoplasma and fungi) which may have more diffuse effects.

Serum potassium is low, which can be explained by a combination of diuretics and poor diet.

b) The investigation of choice would be a laparotomy and removal of the ovaries for histology. Generally a total abdominal hysterectomy is performed, with sampling of the pelvic lymph nodes to stage the disease.

Paraneoplastic cerebellar–brainstem degeneration is most commonly associated with carcinoma of the ovary. Other tumours linked to the syndrome are breast, lung and Hodgkin's disease.

The central nervous system paraneoplastic syndromes tend to overlap with each other. The major groups include:

1) Cerebellar degeneration
2) Limbic encephalitis (amnesia, hallucinations and epilepsy)
3) Lower brainstem encephalitis
4) Spinal cord disease causing a pyramidal or extrapyramidal syndrome
5) Degeneration of the dorsal root ganglia causing a sensory ataxia or anterior horn cell degeneration which may lead to a bulbar palsy.

How certain tumours cause selective neuronal death is not known. Antibodies to cells in the dorsal root ganglia and Purkinje cells have been identified, an observation consistent with an immunological mechanism. Treatment of paraneoplastic CNS-degenerations is rarely effective. Occasionally, removal of the primary neoplasm is followed by improvement.

66 A

a) Marked elevation in the KCO (NB this has been corrected for the Hb) suggesting **alveolar haemorrhage**, which can occur in the absence of frank haemoptysis.

b) Goodpasture's syndrome, Wegener's granulomatosis, microscopic polyarteritis, systemic lupus erythematosus.

B

a) Asthma.

67 a) The clinical presentation is typical of **diaphragmatic weakness**.

This diagnosis should be considered when patients present with shortness of breath which is most marked in the supine position.

This patient has bilateral idiopathic diaphragmatic nerve palsy. Unilateral palsy is much more common, and can also present in this way. Unilateral weakness may be caused by a tumour, particularly bronchial malignancy.

Bilateral diaphragmatic weakness is caused by the following: 1) diseases which affect the C3 to C5 roots in the cervical spine (spinal cord transection, tumour, infection); 2) myopathies and myasthenia gravis (e.g. muscular dystrophy, inflammatory or metabolic myopathies, such as acid maltase deficiency); 3) Herpes zoster infection.

b) Pulmonary function tests in erect and supine positions, fluoroscopic evaluation of diaphragmatic movement, and, if available, phrenic nerve conduction studies, are required. Maximal inspiratory pressures (MIPs) are abnormal, and supine FVC is lower than in the erect position. The paralyzed diaphragm may be elevated on a PA chest X-ray, and dynamic fluoroscopic examination may demonstrate upward movement of the affected diaphragm during sniffing.

Answer to questions 68–69

panarteritis of unknown aetiology affecting large and medium-sized vessels. In most centres it is clinical practice to perform a temporal artery biopsy to confirm the diagnosis before commencing the patient on high-dose corticosteroids. Typically symptoms respond promptly to high doses of prednisolone and this is mirrored by a fall in the acute-phase response. In this case the patient failed to respond to treatment, which raises the possibility of a **paraneoplastic musculoskeletal syndrome**. These may take many forms and include myopathy, arthropathy, polymyalgia, giant-cell arteritis, scleroderma, polymyositis, and vasculitis. Clinically it is impossible to distinguish between true giant-cell arteritis and the paraneoplastic syndrome, but paraneoplastic syndromes tend to respond poorly to conventional doses of prednisolone.

b) A renal cell carcinoma needs to be excluded if the patient has haematuria and proteinuria. Renal cell carcinoma (hypernephroma) has a peak incidence in the 5th to 7th decades and occurs in males more commonly than females.

Renal cell carcinoma may have protean manifestations which include haematuria (55%), elevated ESR (55%), abdominal mass (45%), loin pain (41%), hypertension (35%), weight loss, fever, hypercalcaemia, erythrocytosis and musculoskeletal paraneoplastic syndromes.

69 a) Buerger's disease (thromboangiitis obliterans). This does not occur exclusively in males. Patients from southern Europe are amongst the heaviest smokers in the world, and often smoke unfiltered cigarettes with a high tar content.

b) The diagnosis may be confirmed by Doppler ultrasound of the peripheral vasculature, with a view to proceeding with digital subtraction angiography. The radiographic features of Buerger's disease are characteristic with 'corkscrew' collaterals.

The patient needs a blood film, iron studies, and haemoglobin electrophoresis. Her microcytic anaemia is due to iron deficiency secondary to menorrhagia. Thalassaemia should be excluded in a Mediterranean patient with microcytic anaemia. In addition an iron deficiency anaemia in a patient of 44 years may require gastrointestinal examination. If symptoms are referrable to the upper gastrointestinal tract, an upper GI endoscopy is the first examination. Colonoscopy or barium enema should be considered if the upper GI examination is negative, or if the patient complains of stool blood or change in bowel habit.

c) There are some features which may suggest primary antiphospholipid syndrome and SLE but neither diagnosis is supported by the investigations.

70 This patient is in **cardiogenic shock.**

a) The cyanosis in the presence of fully saturated arterial blood arises from poor peripheral perfusion.

b) Blood flow (cardiac output) is poor and therefore there is greater than normal oxygen extraction at the tissues from each passage of blood through the capillary beds. Inferior vena cava blood is always of lower saturation because hepatic venous blood is extremely desaturated.

c) The high V-wave in the PCWP suggests some mitral regurgitation. This is probably secondary to left ventricular dilation and dysfunction, in which case there is no benefit from surgery. If, however, there is primary mitral valve disease (e.g. damage due to endocarditis) there may be considerable haemodynamic improvement from mitral valve replacement.

d) The arterial blood is fully saturated. The high wedge pressure in the absence of pulmonary arterial hypertension suggests that the pulmonary venous hypertension is relatively acute, and should cause severe pulmonary oedema at this level. The maintenance of full saturation therefore suggests that the patient is receiving inspired oxygen therapy.

Answer to question 71

71 a) Primary biliary cirrhosis. The patient presents with a
cholestatic hepatitis, hepatosplenomegaly, and an upper
gastrointestinal haemorrhage. In addition she has an elevated
serum IgM and her calcium is at the lower limit of normal
(corrected Ca 2.0 mmol/l for an albumin) with a low serum
phosphate suggesting early osteomalacia. Patients with primary
biliary cirrhosis tend to have few stigmata of chronic liver
disease compared with alcoholic liver disease or chronic active
hepatitis.

b) Further investigations should include upper GI endoscopy
to distinguish between a peptic ulcer and bleeding varices
(enlarged spleen suggests portal hypertension),
anti-mitochondrial antibodies and a liver biopsy to confirm the
diagnosis of primary biliary cirrhosis, and vitamin D level to
evaluate the low calcium.

Primary biliary cirrhosis chiefly affects females between 30 and
60 years of age, and is second only to alcohol as a cause of
chronic liver disease in such patients. Primary biliary cirrhosis
may present with deranged liver function tests, pruritus,
jaundice, abdominal pain, anorexia, weight loss, diarrhoea,
osteopenia (and bone pain), and evidence of liver failure or upper
GI bleeding (increased incidence of peptic ulceration).
Xanthelasma are common and chronic cases may be clubbed.
The natural history is variable: asymptomatic patients may never
develop significant disease. Symptomatic patients, e.g. those
who present with pruritus, generally progress to cirrhosis with
portal hypertension over 7–10 years. Why some patients have a
non-progressive form of primary biliary cirrhosis is unknown.

The alkaline phosphatase and γ-GT are raised in >99% of
patients; the alanine transaminase and aspartate amino-
transferase are usually normal. Bilirubin rises late and suggests a
poor prognosis. An elevated IgM is found in 80%, IgG in 40% and
IgA only rarely.

Antimitochondrial antibodies are positive in >90% of cases; the
titre does not have prognostic significance; only four
antimitochondrial antibodies, M2, M4, M8 (associated with a
worse prognosis) and anti-M9 are associated with primary biliary
cirrhosis. Anti-smooth muscle antibody or a weakly positive
antinuclear factor are also common. A strongly positive anti-
smooth muscle antibody or ANA is associated with disease with
features of both chronic active Lupoid hepatitis and primary
biliary cirrhosis.

Histologically the disease is patchy. The earliest lesion is a
T-cell mediated focal damage to the interlobular bile ducts with
associated granuloma formation, followed by bile duct
obliteration/proliferation, fibrosis and finally cirrhosis.

Pruritus may be treated with cholestyramine, antihistamines, or
if these fail, rifampicin or UV-radiation; rarely, haemoperfusion is
necessary. Liver transplantation is now firmly established as
treatment for end-stage primary biliary cirrhosis. D-penicillamine
[Answer continues overleaf]

may produce an improvement in the short term but it is not sustained. Prednisolone improves the biochemical picture but increases osteopenia, hence should only be used with caution. Osteomalacia may be prevented with calcium and vitamin D supplements. Occasionally the other fat-soluble vitamins are reduced and cause symptoms — vitamin K (bruising), vitamin E (neuropathy), and vitamin A (night blindness). High cholesterol levels will require dietary modification.

72 a) A megaloblastic anaemia caused by failure of B_{12} absorption is the most likely diagnosis. The patient has previously undergone emergency surgery for abdominal pain and peritonism, raising the possibility of small bowel resection and/or the blind loop syndrome.

The first part of the Schilling test demonstrates malabsorption of vitamin B_{12}. The purpose of the second part of the test is to assess whether this defect is reversed by simultaneous administration of intrinsic factor. Correction of the malabsorption by intrinsic factor is almost diagnostic of pernicious anaemia. Failure of intestinal absorption is indicated if intrinsic factor fails to reverse the defect.

In blind loop syndromes, B_{12} deficiency is caused by bacterial utilization; the bacteria synthesize folate and the low B_{12} is often matched by a paradoxically high serum folate level.

b) Further investigations should include: i) a small-bowel enema to exclude fistulae, strictures and blind loops, ii) quantitative bacterial analysis on jejunal aspirates and iii) a bile acid breath test.

Bile acid breath test — a radiolabelled ^{14}C conjugated bile acid is given orally and the amount of radioactive carbon dioxide excreted in the breath is measured along with faecal radioactivity. In normal individuals the conjugated bile acid is reabsorbed intact in the terminal ileum and little deconjugation occurs. In bacterial overgrowth affecting the small intestine, the bile acid is rapidly deconjugated and radioactive CO_2 excreted in the breath.

In disease of the terminal ileum, the bile acid is not absorbed and enters the colon where colonic bacteria deconjugate it, leading to radioactive CO_2 production. In ileal disease, unlike bacterial overgrowth, faecal excretion of radioactivity is high. Causes of B_{12} deficiency include:

1) *Nutritional causes*
   Vegans
2) *Gastric causes*
   Addisonian pernicious anaemia, congenital deficiency of intrinsic factor, gastrectomy (partial or total) and atrophic gastritis.
3) *Intestinal causes*
   Blind loop syndrome, ileal resection, Crohn's disease, tropical sprue, fish tapeworm, transcobalamin 11 deficiency.
4) *Drugs*
   Para-aminosalicylic acid, colchicine, alcohol, biguanides.

73 a) The tiredness and cold peripheries are likely to be related to the β-**blocker**, which needs to be either reduced or slowly withdrawn. The fluid retention is caused by the **oestrogen effect of fosfestrol**, which is metabolized to stilboestrol. The high T4 is likely to reflect high thyroxine binding globulin levels induced by stilboestrol. Thyrotoxicosis with symptoms suppressed by atenolol is not likely since the TSH is still within the normal range.

b) Measurement of thyroid binding globulin and the free T4 would be the most appropriate investigations.

74 a) i) **Sub-arachnoid haemorrhage.**
   ii) Meningitis.
Subarachnoid haemorrhage (SAH) is most likely. The patient gives a history of a headache of acute onset — typical of subarachnoid haemorrhage — and is apyrexial.

b) Lumbar puncture (provided no evidence of raised intracranial pressure).
Organisms and/or an elevated WBC and low glucose count point to a diagnosis of meningitis; frankly bloody fluid or xanthochromia (if the tap is performed after 24–48 hours) indicate subarachnoid haemorrhage.
Note: 48 hours after a subarachnoid haemorrhage there may be a reactive cerebrospinal fluid leucocytosis and low sugar.

c) CT scan when possible, full blood count, plasma glucose, clotting profile, blood cultures, CSF culture, routine urea and electrolytes.

d) Ruptured intracranial aneurysm. The commonest sites are the anterior communicating artery 30%, middle carotid artery 25% and posterior communicating 25%; 15% have multiple aneurysms; 5% bleed from arteriovenous malformations.

e) Acutely — the exclusion of meningitis, rest, analgesia ± antiemetic agents, careful monitoring of neurological state, and control of BP are important.
   Diagnosis can be made by CT scanning if available, but lumbar puncture is always indicated if there is any suspicion of meningitis. Referral to a neurosurgical centre for angiography is indicated — rebleeds commonly occur at around 1 week, and may be fatal. If technically possible, surgical clipping of an aneurysm is performed. If no lesion is identified at angiography, management is conservative.

75 a) The differential diagnosis of a unilateral mass on the chest X-ray and a slowly progressive paraparesis would include primary chest carcinoma with spinal secondaries, lymphoma with spinal deposits, infection, e.g. tuberculosis, and sarcoidosis. The elevated serum calcium and low corrected transfer factor favour a diagnosis of **sarcoidosis**, though malignancy cannot be excluded. The hypochromic microcytic anaemia can be explained by the patient's menorrhagia.

b) As a matter of urgency a thoracic myelogram should be performed to exclude cord compression. Other relevant investigations are:

Neurological tests: CT head scan, NMR scans of head, cervical and thoracic spine, CSF examination.

Tests to obtain a tissue diagnosis: CT chest scan, fibreoptic bronchoscopy combined with biopsy or lavage, anterior mediastinoscopy and node biopsy.

Miscellaneous: Serum angiotensin-converting enzyme and Kveim test, serum iron and total iron binding capacity.

In this patient the diagnosis of sarcoidosis was confirmed by finding non-caseating granulomas on blind mucosal biopsy and on lymph node biopsy at mediastinoscopy. The thoracic myelogram and head CT scan were normal but NMR scans showed extensive confluent areas of high signal from the periventricular areas of the brain and upper cervical cord, suggestive of neurosarcoidosis.

Neurosarcoidosis complicates 5% of cases of sarcoidosis and may be the presenting manifestation of sarcoidosis in these patients. Neurosarcoidosis may have protean manifestations and can present with new clinical signs over a prolonged period of time and hence may mimic multiple sclerosis.

Neurosarcoidosis for simplicity may be divided into:
i) neuropathies involving cranial and/or peripheral nerves (VII most commonly involved), and ii) CNS sarcoidosis involving the meninges, brain and spinal cord.

Symptoms and signs include epilepsy, raised intracranial pressure, hypothalamic syndromes, low grade meningitis, pyramidal signs, brainstem syndromes. Sarcoid granulomatous infiltrates in the cervical cord tend to affect primarily the pyramidal tracts.

Prognostically, cases of neurosarcoidosis can be divided into two groups: i) those with a monophasic illness who tend to respond well to high-dose prednisolone and have a good outcome, and ii) those with a chronic or relapsing course, in general responding poorly to prednisolone.

Note: i) Oligoclonal bands may be found in the CSF of cases of neurosarcoidosis; ii) 2% of patients with sarcoidosis have unilateral hilar lymphadenopathy.

76 A

a) A glucagonoma. Glucagonomas are alpha-cell pancreatic tumours which secrete glucagon and other related pancreatic peptides. They are present in adult life and are more common in females than males. Patients typically present with a necrolytic migratory rash and diabetes mellitus; other features include weight loss, diarrhoea and venous thrombosis.

b) The diagnosis is confirmed by finding elevated fasting plasma glucagon levels.

c) Surgical excision is the treatment of choice, and if removal is complete, is associated with complete resolution of symptoms. Many of these tumours are, however, widely disseminated at the time of diagnosis. Streptozotocin may be used to reduce metastasis size and symptoms; arterial embolization may be used to treat hepatic secondaries. The diabetes is usually insulin-dependent, anticoagulation will reduce the risk of thrombosis and oral zinc supplements may help the rash.

B

a) Primary hyperaldosteronism — Conn's syndrome — due to an adrenal adenoma or adrenal hyperplasia. The combination of hypertension with the biochemical picture of hypernatraemia, hypokalaemia and a high serum bicarbonate concentration is typical. Hypertension and hypokalaemic alkalosis are also seen with ectopic ACTH production but the glucose level is usually elevated.

b) The diagnosis is confirmed by high serum aldosterone levels in the presence of low renin levels. The hypertension is typically resistant to ACE inhibitors. Arteriography and venous sampling, CT scanning, and cholesterol scanning are used to localize the source of aldosterone prior to surgery.

77 a) The disorder is **familial hypophosphataemic rickets**, inherited in an **X-linked dominant manner**. Tubular resorption of phosphate is defective, leading to low plasma phosphate levels. Phosphate deficiency is the primary cause of the osteomalacia, which is characterized in these patients by a raised ALP but usually a normal or minimally-reduced plasma calcium concentration. Since the calcium is relatively normal there is rarely evidence of hyperparathyroidism. The diagnosis may be confirmed by showing an inappropriate phosphaturia. Treatment is large doses of phosphate and if necessary a small dose of vitamin D.

b) A has a 50% chance of being affected.
   B will be unaffected (mother has two normal X chromosomes).

78 The combination of acute onset neurological abnormalities in association with microangiopathic haemolytic anaemia, disseminated intravascular coagulation, thrombocytopenia, and renal failure is highly suggestive of **thrombotic thrombocytopenic purpura.**

Thrombotic thrombocytopenic purpura is a disorder of unknown aetiology which primarily affects young females. Typically there is sudden onset of fever, neurological signs, evidence of bleeding and renal failure of varying severity. It is closely related to the haemolytic uraemic syndrome of childhood, though neurological involvement is much commoner. Pathophysiologically the initial event is believed to be blood vessel endothelial cell damage which subsequently triggers the clotting cascade leading to platelet consumption and fibrin deposition, the latter damaging red blood cells producing the classical fragmented or helmet cells. Histologically there is widespread evidence of microvascular hyaline thrombi.

Treatment is difficult; in view of the grave prognosis, corticosteroids, immunosuppressive agents, immunoglobulin infusions and plasma exchange have been used with varying success. Anticoagulation is sometimes judiciously used in an effort to halt the consumptive coagulopathy, its possible beneficial effects being balanced against the risk of haemorrhage.

Microangiopathic haemolytic anaemia describes the mechanical destruction of red blood cells in small blood vessels which arises secondary to changes which include microthrombi, fibrinoid necrosis and malignant cell infiltration. The blood film typically shows microspherocytes and fragmented red cells. Many patients with a microangiopathic haemolytic anaemia also have evidence of disseminated intravascular coagulation but the two disorders may occur separately and do not necessarily overlap. A reduced platelet count suggests an associated disseminated intravascular coagulation.

Causes of microangiopathic haemolytic anaemia include:

Septicaemia — e.g. meningococcal septicaemia
Haemolytic uraemic syndrome
Thrombotic thrombocytopenic purpura
Malignant hypertension
Pre-eclampsia
Renal cortical necrosis
Acute glomerulonephritis
Disseminated mucinous carcinomatosis
Polyarteritis nodosa
Wegener's granulomatosis
SLE

79 a) No. Pulmonary oedema will usually occur when pulmonary venous pressure exceeds 25 mmHg. Orthopnoea will occur at lower pressures, therefore this patient will experience breathlessness on lying flat.

b) i) Ventriculoseptal defect.
   ii) Acute mitral regurgitation.

c) Measurement of oxygen saturation of blood from the right atrial and pulmonary arterial ports of the Swan–Ganz catheter. If there is a ventriculoseptal defect the pulmonary artery blood will be significantly more saturated than right atrial blood.

d) Inspiration causes a reduction in intrathoracic pressure. The pulmonary veins are exclusively intrathoracic and inspiration will reduce pulmonary venous pressure and aid pulmonary venous return. Left ventricular stroke volume will be reduced and hence the flow of blood either across the mitral valve or ventriculoseptal defect in systole will be reduced, leading to a reduction in murmur intensity.

80 a) This man has evidence of **pituitary failure**, possibly as a result of his head injury. He has a low T4 but no compensatory rise in TSH; he has lost axillary and pubic hair, suggesting hypogonadism; he is pale, has a low sodium and postural hypotension features of ACTH deficiency.
Note: ACTH deficiency does not cause significant hyponatraemia, so typical of primary adrenal failure, since aldosterone is still secreted normally. There is however a dilutional hyponatraemia and postural hypotension due to cortisol deficiency.

b) Investigations should include: i) measurement of pituitary hormones (TSH, ACTH, FSH, LH, GH, PRL), ii) measurement of other target hormones (T4, testosterone and cortisol), iii) a CT head scan to image the pituitary fossa, and iv) dynamic pituitary function tests to distinguish between pituitary and hypothalamic dysfunction (insulin-induced hypoglycaemia, and administration of TRH and GnRH).

c) Replacement therapy consists of hydrocortisone, oral thyroxine and depot testosterone. Thyroid replacement should be introduced under careful supervision in view of the history of ischaemic heart disease. Thyroxine should be started in low dosage and there is an argument for initially starting liothyronine in view of its shorter half life should angina be precipitated. An explanation of the patient's therapy should emphasize that the treatment is for life and that the cortisol dose should be increased during illness.

81 a) The commonest cause of a Coombs'-negative haemolytic anaemia is **hereditary spherocytosis** (an autosomal dominant disorder).

Haemolysis is indicated by reticulocytosis, absent haptoglobins and a raised bilirubin. The history suggestive of recurrent haemolysis, the family history of anaemia and splenomegaly are all compatible with this diagnosis.

The blood film shows microspherocytes and the diagnosis may be confirmed by demonstrating the increased red cell osmotic fragility caused by the hereditary red cell membrane abnormality.

A full family study should then be performed on the direct relatives of patients with this disorder. Splenectomy is usually performed in all cases, though it is usually delayed until 5 years of age because of the increased risk of infection (especially pneumococcal). Prophylactic daily penicillin and pneumococcal vaccination are recommended post-splenectomy.

82 a) A right deep venous thrombosis consequent upon **paroxysmal nocturnal haemoglobinuria.**

  b) i) A right venogram.

  ii) Ham's test (acid lysis test), which measures the sensitivity of red blood cells to complement lysis.

The occurrence of a thrombotic episode in a patient with pancytopenia is highly suggestive of paroxysmal nocturnal haemoglobinuria (PNH). In this patient PNH is also suggested by the history of dark urine passed early in the morning, and intermittent abdominal pain. PNH is an acquired clonal disorder characterized by a membrane abnormality which results in increased sensitivity to complement. It sometimes develops during the recovery phase of an acute aplastic anaemia. Clinically there is intermittent, classically nocturnal, haemolysis leading to dark urine. The haemolysis may be profound and life threatening. The mechanism of the thrombotic tendency is not clear but may reflect the susceptibility of platelets to complement activation. Other important sites for thrombosis include hepatic vein obstruction, producing the Budd–Chiari syndrome, and cerebral thrombosis. The episodes of abdominal pain are thought to result from episodes of thrombosis affecting small portal blood vessels.

The severity of the symptoms varies; some patients require regular blood transfusions. Corticosteroids and androgens have been used in an effort to control the degree of haemolysis, and iron supplements are necessary as a result of the considerable haemosiderinuria. Anticoagulation is necessary for thrombotic episodes. In some patients the condition is self-limiting as the abnormal clone disappears. Allogeneic bone marrow transplantation has been successfully performed in patients with severe disease.

83 a) Primary adrenal failure — the biochemical picture of hyponatraemia, hyperkalaemia, a moderately increased urea, and hypoglycaemia is typical. Moderate corrected hypercalcaemia is also a recognized feature of adrenal failure.

The low T4 raises the possibility of secondary adrenal failure but the increased TSH indicates normal pituitary function. A low T4 and high TSH are frequently seen in Addison's disease in the absence of functional hypothyroidism, and revert to normal following steroid replacement.

Addison's disease in the Western world is most commonly autoimmune in nature and is associated with autoimmune hypothyroidism in approximately 10% of cases. In this case, the absence of thyroid antibodies and the patient's race puts tuberculosis higher on the list of causes of adrenal failure. The diagnosis may be confirmed by:

1) The short synacthen test — 250 mg of tetracosactrin is administered followed by measurement of cortisol levels at 0, 30 and 60 minutes. Failure of cortisol to increase by 250 nmol/l at 30 minutes to a level greater than 550 nmol/l confirms the diagnosis.
2) Measurement of ACTH levels — elevated in primary adrenal failure.
3) Abdominal X-ray — evidence of adrenal calcification with tuberculous adrenal destruction.
4) Measurement of adrenal autoantibodies.

b) Glucocorticoid replacement, typically hydrocortisone 20 mg in the morning and 10 mg at night. Mineralocorticoid replacement with fludrocortisone 0.1 mg o.d. may be necessary.

84 a) Coronary artery atherosclerosis. ST segment depression extending from lead V3 to V6 of greater than 2 mm suggests ischaemia in the region supplied by the left anterior descending artery.

b) The QRS complexes in the V leads demonstrate the voltage criteria for left ventricular hypertrophy. In the absence of systemic hypertension, aortic stenosis must be considered. This may cause exercise-induced ischaemia without coronary artery disease.

c) i)   Echocardiography to exclude aortic stenosis.
   ii)   Coronary arteriography.

85 a An incomplete urine collection.

In this patient, at first glance the Schilling test is suggestive of terminal ileal Crohn's disease as the cause of the malabsorption — the addition of intrinsic factor does not increase B_{12} absorption. However, the urinary creatinine is too low for a male of average weight with grossly normal renal function. The calculated glomerular filtration rate from the above figures is 60.

$$GFR = \frac{[Creatinine]\ urine \times 24\ hour\ urine\ vol}{[Creatinine]\ plasma \times 1440} = 60\ ml/min$$

A glomerular filtration rate of 60 ml/min is compatible with a normal serum urea and creatinine but strongly suggests that the patient has only collected approximately 50% of his 24-hour urine output.

The $^{14}CO_2$ breath test provides confirmatory evidence that the low B_{12} is due to bacterial overgrowth and not terminal ileal disease.

86 A

a) The severe microcytosis in the absence of anaemia in a patient of appropriate ethnic origin is highly suggestive of either alpha or beta thalassaemia cell trait. The elevated Hb A2 >3.5% and Hb F are diagnostic of **beta thalassaemia trait.** Haemoglobin electrophoresis is normal in cases of alpha thalassaemia and alpha/beta chain synthesis ratio studies are needed for diagnosis.

b) The patient should be reassured that he will remain entirely asymptomatic. However it is vitally important that he and his partner are counselled about the implications of parenthood; if they are planning to have children his partner should be investigated for thalassaemia trait. If both are beta thalassaemia trait positive there is a 25% chance that one of their offspring will have beta thalassaemia major; this can be detected antenatally.

B

a) Chronic renal failure. Chronic renal failure explains the mild hyperkalaemia and acidosis, the hypocalcaemia and the normochromic normocytic anaemia. Most patients with chronic renal failure will have a low T4 and T3 but a normal TSH and TRH response. The T4 tends to normalize once effective renal replacement therapy is introduced.

Causes of galactorrhoea include:

1) Pregnancy
2) Antidopaminergic drugs — phenothiazines, butyrophenones, metoclopramide, methyldopa
3) Oestrogens
4) Hypothalamic/pituitary lesions
5) Hypothyroidism
6) Chronic renal failure
7) Ectopic prolactin secretion, e.g. bronchogenic carcinoma, hypernephroma.

87 A

a) The clinical picture is one of a right femoral nerve lesion in a patient with a prolonged prothrombin time. The most likely diagnosis is a **psoas bleed** causing **femoral nerve compression** due to **over-anticoagulation** with **warfarin**. The recent change in drug treatment is the most likely culprit — amiodarone typically potentiates the effect of warfarin.

The diagnosis of a psoas bleed may be confirmed by ultrasound or CT scan. The coagulopathy should urgently be reversed by infusion of fresh frozen plasma. Vitamin K is a competitive antagonist of warfarin and will correct the prolonged prothrombin time. However, vitamin K is contraindicated in a patient with a prosthetic valve since it may be difficult to re-anticoagulate for several days.

B

a) The presence of a macrocytic anaemia, neutropenia and thrombocytopenia suggests a diagnosis of **myelodysplasia**. This diagnosis is supported by the presence of Pelger cells and circulating blasts. It is now recognized that there is a 7–10-fold increase in the incidence of acute myeloid leukaemia after intensive chemotherapy for Hodgkin's disease. These leukaemias are usually preceded by myelodysplasia. The risk of developing leukaemia is greatest 5 years after treatment but remains high for up to 8 years after the last course of chemotherapy. An increased risk of acute myeloid leukaemia also occurs in other diseases such as myeloma, polycythaemia rubra vera and carcinoma of the ovary and breast where alkylating agents are used. Such secondary leukaemias are associated with particular karyotypes such as 5q–. The long arm of chromosome 5 encodes a series of haemopoietic growth factors and differentiation antigens, and its deletion raises fascinating questions concerning the mechanism of secondary leukaemia.

Immunosuppression with non-alkylating agents, as in recipients of renal or cardiac transplantation, is associated with an increased risk of non-Hodgkin's lymphoma.

88 a) There is an obvious delta wave which is positive in lead V1. This is **Wolff–Parkinson–White syndrome type A.**

b) i)   A re-entrant supraventricular tachycardia.
    ii)   Atrial fibrillation.

The danger of atrial fibrillation is that the accessory path may be capable of conducting very fast atrial rates, leading to a fast ventricular response which may degenerate into ventricular arrhythmias.

c) Posterior myocardial infarction
    Right bundle branch block
    Right ventricular hypertrophy
    Dextrocardia
    Duchenne's muscular dystrophy.

89 A

a) Autoimmune haemolytic anaemia complicating chronic lymphatic leukaemia. The presence of lymphocytosis with lymphadenopathy and splenomegaly in this age group is very suggestive of chronic lymphatic leukaemia. Anaemia in chronic lymphatic leukaemia may be caused by marrow infiltration, hypersplenism or an autoimmune haemolytic anaemia. In this patient the polychromasia, spherocytosis, reticulocytosis and absent haptoglobins point to a diagnosis of haemolysis.

b) Direct Coombs' test. About 20% of patients with chronic lymphatic leukaemia will develop a positive Coombs' test at some time during their illness but only one-third will develop significant haemolysis.

The haemolysis responds well to steroids and chlorambucil.

B

a) The coagulation tests show a prolonged activated partial thromboplastin time (APTT) but normal prothrombin time (PT), indicating an abnormality of the intrinsic pathway of coagulation. The commonest cause of such an abnormality is factor VIII:C deficiency — **haemophilia A**, an X-linked recessive condition.

Factor IX deficiency — Haemophilia B/Christmas disease (X-linked R) — will also produce the same abnormal clotting profile but its incidence is one-fifth that of haemophilia A.

b) Severe factor VIII deficiency (<1% normal levels) causes impaired generation of thrombin and results in bleeding into major weight-bearing joints and prolonged bleeding after surgery or dental extraction. Intracranial bleeding is the commonest cause of death in severe untreated haemophilia; other common sites of bleeding include the renal tract, muscles, subperiosteal region and the iliopsoas sheath. The severity of symptoms depends on the extent of factor VIII:C deficiency.

Primary haemostasis, which is caused by a combination of vasoconstriction and platelet aggregation, is normal in haemophilia A and B and there is no abnormality in the initial haemostatic response. The diagnosis may be confirmed by demonstrating a deficiency of factor VIII:C and normal levels of factor IX and X.

Note: In von Willebrand's disease (autosomal D inheritance) abnormal platelet function is associated with low factor VIII:C and VIIIR:AG activity. The following tests are abnormal: prolonged APTT (may be normal), prolonged bleeding time and impaired ristocetin-induced platelet aggregation.

90 a) Primary hyperparathyroidism — approximately 83% of cases are due to a single adenoma; diffuse gland hyperplasia accounts for approximately 10% and multiple adenoma for 4% of cases.

Investigations show hypercalcaemia, a low phosphate, a raised alkaline phosphatase, and a hyperchloraemic metabolic acidosis. The elevated blood urea may be explained by dehydration subsequent to the polyuria induced by the hypercalcaemia. There is a well-recognized association between primary hyperparathyroidism and peptic ulceration, which explains the epigastric pain (note: a gastrointestinal bleed could also account for the elevated urea).

b) Most patients with primary hyperparathyroidism are diagnosed on routine screening and are asymptomatic.

Clinical features include abdominal pain, renal colic, constipation, vomiting, polydipsia, polyuria, weakness, psychiatric changes, band keratopathy, peptic ulceration and pancreatitis. Fifty percent of patients with primary hyperparathyroidism will develop renal stones.

Note the association of i) primary hyperparathyroidism, pituitary tumours, pancreatic tumours and adrenal cortical tumours — multiple-endocrine neoplasia type I (MEN Type I), and ii) primary hyperparathyroidism, medullary carcinoma of the thyroid, phaeochromocytomas, carcinoid tumours and mucosal neuromas (MEN Type II).

c) The diagnosis is confirmed by finding an inappropriately high parathyroid hormone level for the serum calcium. Other features of primary hyperparathyroidism include:

1) a hyperchloraemic metabolic acidosis (unlike other cases of hypercalcaemia)
2) elevated 24-hour urinary calcium excretion
3) elevated urinary cAMP
4) elevated urinary hydroxyproline excretion
5) radiology: subperiosteal bone resorption, bone cysts, brown tumours and deformities
6) the hydrocortisone suppression test fails to suppress calcium levels in primary hyperparathyroidism but does so in other cases of hypercalcaemia.

d) Causes of hypercalcaemia include:

1) Malignancy
2) Multiple myeloma
3) Primary hyperparathyroidism
4) Tertiary hyperparathyroidism
5) Sarcoidosis
6) Vitamin D toxicity
7) Milk–alkali syndrome
8) Hyperthyroidism
9) Adrenal failure
10) Immobility with Paget's disease
11) Phaeochromocytoma
12) Thiazide diuretics.

91 a) Polymyositis is the most likely diagnosis despite the normal muscle biopsy. Criteria for the diagnosis of polymyositis include:
1) symmetrical proximal muscle weakness
2) typical EMG changes
3) typical muscle biopsy
4) elevated serum muscle enzymes
5) skin changes of dermatomyositis.

Difficulty in climbing stairs is an early symptom of proximal muscle weakness and this is often accompanied by pain and stiffness.

Muscle enzymes (aspartate amino-transferase and creatinine phosphokinase) are raised and the EMG changes are typical. Approximately 20% of muscle biopsies are negative as the disease is often patchy in its distribution.

The erythrocyte sedimentation rate and serum immunoglobulins are often elevated, as in this case.

The autoantibodies anti-Jo1, anti-P17 and anti-Pl12 are found in a subset of polymyositis patients who develop pulmonary fibrosis.

Clinical investigations to detect occult malignancy should be considered in patients over the age of 50.

92 a) Investigation was performed during the investigation of suspected **acromegaly.**

b) Two diagnoses may be made:
i) the patient is acromegalic: baseline growth hormone levels are elevated and fail to suppress with an oral glucose tolerance test.
ii) the patient is also diabetic.

Whole blood glucose values are 10–15% less than plasma. Capillary values are approximately 8% greater than venous values.

Diagnostic values for 750 g oral glucose tolerance test (in 250 ml water)

Venous whole blood	Fasting mmol/l	Two hours post oral GTT mmol/l
Normal	<6.7	<6.7
Diabetes mellitus	≥6.7	≥10
Impaired glucose tolerance	<6.7	>6.7 ≤10
Venous plasma	Fasting mmol/l	Two hours post oral GTT mmol/l
Normal	<7.8	<7.8
Diabetes mellitus	≥7.8	≥11.1
Impaired glucose tolerance	<7.8	>7.8 ≤11.1

93 A

a) Aluminium toxicity.

b) First stop aluminium hydroxide, and use a non-aluminium-containing phosphate binder as necessary. Definitive treatment involves intravenous desferrioxamine. Patients with end-stage renal failure are at risk of aluminium toxicity for the following reasons: i) renal excretion of the element is impaired, ii) dialysate is a source of additional aluminium, and iii) aluminium hydroxide is often used as a phosphate binder. Aluminium accumulates in the bone, liver, spleen, brain, muscles, heart and parathyroid glands. Aluminium toxicity produces two main clinical patterns:

1) dialysis dementia, characterized by personality change, dyspraxia, speech disturbance, myoclonic jerks and global dementia.
2) aluminium bone disease, characterized by bone pain, diffuse demineralization and secondary fractures. Biochemically, serum calcium levels are normal or raised and serum PTH undetectable.

Diagnosis is made by measurement of serum aluminium levels, though these tend to reflect recent exposure and the rise in serum aluminium level during a desferrioxamine infusion provides more useful information. Bone biopsy remains the definitive diagnostic test.

B

a) The cerebellum.

b) The combination of polycythaemia and cerebellar signs suggests a diagnosis of von Hippel–Lindau syndrome. The syndrome is inherited in an autosomal dominant fashion. Haemangioblastomas develop throughout the central nervous system but show a predilection for the cerebellum. Von Hippel–Lindau syndrome is one of the recognized causes of ectopic erythropoietin production. Other recognized features include: i) cysts affecting the kidney, liver and pancreas, ii) renal cell carcinoma, and iii) phaeochromocytoma.

94 a) The biochemical picture is one of a **high anion gap metabolic acidosis**. In the context of the given history the likely cause is **lactic acidosis** subsequent to an inferior myocardial infarction and shock.

The anion gap is an estimation of the total unmeasured plasma anions which in association with HCO_3^- and Cl^- balance plasma cations, which are predominantly Na^+ and K^+ (also Mg^{2+} and Ca^{2+}). The unmeasured plasma anions include proteins, organic acids, Po_4^{2-} and SO_4^{2-}.

For simplicity:

Anion gap = (Na mmol/l + K mmol/l) – (Cl mmol/l + HCO_3 mmol/l).
Anion gap normal range 7–17

In the above example, anion gap = 28 mmol/l.
Measurement of plasma lactate (normally less than 2 mmol/l) would confirm the diagnosis. Measurement of arterial blood gases and pH may be useful in patients of this sort.
Causes of lactic acidosis include:

1) Shock
2) Infection
3) Diabetes mellitus
4) Renal failure
5) Liver failure
6) Drugs, e.g. biguanides — phenformin and metformin, and alcohol
7) Congenital causes, e.g. glucose-6-phosphate dehydrogenase deficiency.

95 a) This M-mode clearly cuts across the mitral valve. **Rheumatic fever** is the only common cause of mitral stenosis.

b) Structure A is the intraventricular septum. Right ventricle is above and left ventricle below the line.

c) The 2 leaflets of the mitral valve separate in diastole; their echo signal is normally a sharp single line each, and they move in opposite directions. B is the posterior leaflet and i) is thickened, and ii) moves anteriorly in diastole (i.e. upwards). This is characteristic of mitral stenosis. In addition the normal pattern of movement of the leaflets is to drift together in mid-diastole and to re-open with atrial contraction. When the left atrial pressure is high they remain open at the limit of their excursion at all times, as shown here.

d) With a mobile stenosed valve, mitral valve opening can be heard as an early diastolic opening snap. This occurs at line C.

96 a) The man has presented with an acute febrile illness characterized by gastrointestinal and respiratory symptoms, unexplained confusion, mild hepatitis, hyponatraemia, hypocalcaemia and relative hypophosphataemia. The most likely diagnosis is **Legionella pneumonia**. Infection with *M. pneumoniae* or an ornithosis may have similar clinical features but would not be expected to produce such a low sodium and calcium.

Legionella occurs sporadically or in epidemics. The natural habitat of *Legionella* species is fresh water; a wide temperature (5–65°C) and pH range (5.5–8.2) is acceptable. Water storage systems such as air-conditioning apparatus, cooling towers and hospital hot water supplies have all been implicated as sources in a variety of epidemics.

Legionnaires' disease typically affects people between 40 and 70 years. There is a high incidence among transplant and other immunosuppressed patients. Abdominal symptoms may dominate the clinical presentation, including pain, diarrhoea and distension; rarely, peritonitis and pancreatitis occur. An enlarged liver and abnormal liver function tests are common. The pneumonia is typically widespread and may heal with fibrosis. In addition to confusion and hallucinations, ataxia, peripheral neuropathy and memory defects may occur. Hyponatraemia, hypocalcaemia, hypophosphataemia and lymphopenia are commonly seen. Haematuria occurs commonly; renal failure is rare. Pericarditis, myocarditis and endocarditis are rare.

b) Investigations should include serology for legionella, mycoplasma, and chlamydia. A bronchoscopy should be performed to obtain material for culture and microscopy (if the condition and pO_2 of the patient permit).

Antibodies start to appear 5–10 days after the onset of symptoms; for definite serological confirmation of legionella infection, comparison of acute and convalescent sera is required. A single sample with a titre of 1/250 or greater is, however, highly suggestive. Culture of the organism requires special conditions and selective media; it grows slowly so that 2–3 weeks may be required to detect the organism in this way. It may be seen on microscopy using silver stains or immunofluorescence.

c) Treatment is either with erythromycin or rifampicin. The prognosis is related to the patient's age, the severity of the pneumonia and the existence of any concomitant disease. Symptoms of poor memory and general irritability may persist for months following recovery.

Chlorination and filtration of water supplies will eliminate the organism.

97 a) The most likely diagnosis is **bacterial endocarditis.**

b) Investigations should include: i) serial cultures of blood and urine, ii) an echocardiogram, and iii) angiography of her left iliac artery. The upper abdominal pain, spleen tenderness and wedge defects are splenic infarcts. The pulsatile left iliac fossa mass is a mycotic aneurysm. The neurological symptoms result from emboli.

In adults nearly a third of cases of infective endocarditis develop on a previously normal valve, and another third occur in patients with mitral valve prolapse. A minority of patients who develop infective endocarditis have a previous history of serious valve disease, e.g. rheumatic fever. Cerebral emboli occur in nearly 20% of cases, typically in the middle cerebral artery territory. The formation of a cerebral mycotic aneurysm is particularly ominous since they have a high chance of rupturing, causing a subarachnoid haemorrhage or intraventricular haemorrhage.

The clinical features of infective endocarditis include fever, evidence of an acute phase response, polyclonal activation of B-cells producing raised rheumatoid factors and a false positive VDRL, petechial haemorrhages, splinter haemorrhages, Osler's nodes (pulp of the finger), Janeway lesions (on the thenar and hypothenar eminence), Roth spots (retinal infarcts), conjunctival haemorrhages, splenomegaly, and in long-standing cases, clubbing. Emboli may affect any organ. Renal lesions include both emboli and glomerulonephritis. Effects on the nervous system reflect embolic phenomena. In chronic cases a normochromic normocytic anaemia develops. The WBC may be raised, normal or in severe cases depressed.

In 90% of cases the organism is grown from blood culture; previous antibiotic administration or unusual organisms account for most of the exceptions. Both *Coxiella burnetti* and mycoplasma may cause endocarditis and can be detected serologically.

The principles of treatment are sterilization of the valve using appropriate antibiotics (usually given for 6 weeks) followed by surgery if the valve is badly damaged. Considerations for early surgery should include infection with organisms such as *Staphylococcus aureus* or *Streptococcus pneumoniae* which are characterized by rapid tissue destruction, fungal endocarditis, patients with aortic root infection, and patients with prosthetic valves.

98 a) Myasthenia gravis. On examination muscle weakness may not be apparent unless strength is examined repeatedly.

b) i) Fatiguability may be demonstrated electrically by repetitive supramaximal stimulation of a suitable peripheral nerve while recording the muscle group evoked potential.

ii) The fatiguability of the affected muscles may be temporarily corrected by edrophonium (Tensilon test).

iii) The disease may be confirmed by detecting antibodies to acetylcholine receptors.

iv) X-ray thoracic inlet

v) CT scan of the neck and chest

vi) Thyroid function tests

vii) Autoantibody profile.

The muscles most often affected are ocular and shoulder girdle. However the muscles of respiration and proximal lower limbs may also be involved early. Breathlessness may develop very quickly and may cause sudden death. Bulbar involvement causes swallowing problems, slurred speech and difficulty chewing. External ocular muscle weakness is often asymmetrical and if a single muscle is affected may mimic a cranial nerve palsy. Pupillary reflexes are always normal. Mild ptosis and weak facial muscles may give the patient a 'snarl' or a depressed look. Eventually muscles of the neck and trunk become involved. Thymic enlargement may be seen in approximately 15% of cases, especially in young patients. In 25% of cases there is evidence of local invasion but not distal spread.

The disease is autoimmune in origin and may be associated with other diseases such as systemic lupus erythematosus, thyrotoxicosis and diabetes mellitus. Thyrotoxicosis may worsen symptoms and signs. Antibodies against acetylcholine receptors on the postsynaptic membrane have a pathogenic role.

Initial treatment is with steroids with or without azathioprine; after improvement has occurred thymectomy should be performed. The benefit of thymectomy cannot be predicted; therefore all cases with generalized disease or thymoma irrespective of age or sex should be offered the operation. Plasmapheresis by removing antibody is a useful short-term measure in severe cases. Anticholinesterase drugs such as pyridostigmine are useful in improving muscle strength.

99 a) The normal left ventricular cavity at end diastole is less than 5.5 cm across; there is therefore cavity dilatation present.

b) 'A' is a sound occurring immediately after the QRS complex of the ECG and must therefore be the first heart sound.

c) The signal occurs in the phase preceding the first heart sound and must be diastolic. The doppler signal is above the centre line, which corresponds to blood flowing towards the transducer at the apex.

d) Diastolic flow across the aortic valve towards the apex can only be **regurgitation**. The left ventricular cavity enlargement is therefore secondary to **aortic incompetence**.

100 a) The most likely diagnosis is **normal pressure hydrocephalus** which is characterized by amnesia (often with psychomotor retardation), gait apraxia and urinary incontinence. There are generally few cortical features such as dysphasia or apraxia, unlike Alzheimer's disease. The onset is typically insidious but may be rapid. There is dilatation of the cerebral ventricles caused by subarachnoid obstruction but normal CSF pressure is recorded if a lumbar puncture is performed.

The syndrome has been observed following head injury, subarachnoid haemorrhage, intracranial surgery, cerebrovascular disease and meningoencephalitis, and in association with lesions which obstruct the third ventricle such as gliomas, cerebellar haemangioblastomas, aqueduct stenosis, third ventricular cysts, and aberrant blood vessels. In 50% of cases there is no clear cause. There is impaired outflow and resorption of CSF; this dilates the ventricles, stretches the periventricular pathways, reduces cerebral blood flow and causes oedema of the periventricular substance. Positron-emission tomography has demonstrated generalized disturbances of cerebral metabolism in normal pressure hydrocephalus as distinct from degenerative diseases.

b) CSF diversion procedures in selected patients can completely reverse the abnormalities (generally ventriculoatrial or ventriculo-peritoneal shunts). It is important to distinguish normal pressure hydrocephalus from the passive ventricular enlargement secondary to cerebral atrophy, which will not benefit from a shunt procedure. CT scanning and intracranial pressure measurement are useful — lack of cortical atrophy and the presence of frontal white matter and periventricular lucency favour normal pressure hydrocephalus. CSF diversion may be complicated by shunt infection, subdural haematomas, epilepsy, and malfunction.

101 a) He has a reduced peak flow, mild hypoxia, and a partially-compensated respiratory alkalosis. These results are consistent with **acute asthma**. Treatment is a high inspired pO_2, bronchodilators (nebulizer or intravenous) and intravenous hydrocortisone. A chest X-ray should be obtained to exclude a concomitant pneumothorax and pneumonia. The response to treatment must be monitored by reassessing his vital signs, the peak flow and blood gases after 1–2 hours.

b) The patient has become more hypoxic and has developed a respiratory acidosis. This is consistent with alveolar hypoventilation. The most important diagnosis to exclude is a pneumothorax. Other causes are impaired respiratory drive (drugs), pneumonia, a collapsed lung (obstruction of a bronchus), and patient exhaustion. Mechanical ventilation should be considered urgently if an easily-reversible cause is not rapidly identified and further deterioration occurs.

102 a) B is a murmur on the phonocardiogram which can be seen from the ECG to be systolic.

b) The aortic root is full of echoes during both systole and diastole. This is due to distortion of the aortic valve. B is therefore an aortic ejection murmur.

c) The structure behind the aortic root is the left atrium. This should not exceed 4.5 cm in diameter. It is thus enlarged according to the 1 cm markers.

d) There is mitral valve disease. There are two reasons from the echocardiogram shown:
i) Rheumatic aortic valve disease never occurs in the absence of mitral valve involvement.
ii) Gross left atrial enlargement (7.5 cm) strongly suggests mitral valve disease.

103 a) The most likely diagnosis is **cystic fibrosis**. The young boy has evidence of malabsorption, chronic respiratory symptoms, a dilated right colon, and is small for his age.

b) Investigations should include a sweat test — the characteristic defect is that secretions contain too little water relative to the protein and electrolyte content, causing mucoviscidosis. A sodium content above 100 mmol/l is consistent with the diagnosis. Other investigations include an assessment of pancreatic function: plasma trypsin and amylase are reduced in chronic pancreatic disease because of loss of cell numbers; an oral glucose tolerance test is useful to assess endocrine pancreatic function. Direct assessment of the pancreas requires measurement of enzymes and bicarbonate in a duodenal aspirate before and after a test meal (the Lundh test); such tests are difficult to perform.

Cystic fibrosis is an autosomal recessive condition, characterized by abnormal exocrine secretion. The major clinical features include chronic pulmonary disease, pancreatic dysfunction resulting in malabsorption, poor growth and diabetes mellitus. The most important problems are respiratory: recurrent bronchiolar obstruction causes bronchiectasis, atelectasis and chronic infection which gradually destroys lung function, ultimately leading to pulmonary insufficiency, and cor pulmonale. Allergic bronchopulmonary aspergillosis is common. The lungs often become colonized by *Staphylococcus pyogenes* and *Pseudomonas aeruginosa*. Hypoplasia of the gall bladder occurs and there is an increased tendency to form gallstones; blockage of bile ducts leads to pericholangitis, periportal fibrosis and biliary cirrhosis. Intestinal problems are related to the secretion of abnormal amounts of viscid mucus and include meconium ileus, intestinal obstruction and reduced transit in the distal bowel.

Treatment is partially successful so that patients now regularly reach adulthood. Physiotherapy and replacement of pancreatic enzymes are the two principal measures. Immunization and the rapid use of antibiotics help to minimize pulmonary damage. Ranitidine is helpful in decreasing the acid digestion of pancreatic enzymes. Genetic counselling should be offered to the parents and other unaffected siblings; prenatal diagnosis is now available.

104 a) The man has progressive breathlessness, without evidence of heart failure or obstructive airways disease, and associated with a positive ANA, latex and raised immunoglobulins (high total protein). The most likely diagnosis is **cryptogenic fibrosing alveolitis**. He also has a mild biochemical hepatitis, seen in 10% of cryptogenic fibrosing alveolitis cases. The raised urea is likely to be caused by diuretics. Since his symptoms had begun before the prescription of amiodarone this is unlikely to have been the original trigger. The main differential diagnoses to consider are:

1) Lung fibrosis associated with a connective tissue disease or vasculitis
2) Extrinsic allergic alveolitis — exposure to organic dusts
3) Bronchiectasis
4) Left sided heart failure
5) Sarcoidosis
6) Lymphangiitis carcinomatosa
7) Pulmonary embolism
8) Industrial lung diseases.

b) Investigations should include pulmonary function tests, including TLCO and KCO estimation to demonstrate lung restriction and reduced gas transfer; a lung biopsy, either open or via a bronchoscope, to establish a histological diagnosis and provide prognostic information. If these results were normal or the lung biopsy showed granulomas then a Kveim test and serum angiotensin-converting enzyme estimation to exclude sarcoidosis should be obtained. Finally a right heart catheter study to measure pulmonary artery pressure should be performed.

The histological features of cryptogenic fibrosing alveolitis include (i) cellular infiltration and fibrosis of the lung parenchyma and (ii) desquamation of altered type II pneumocytes and macrophages into the alveolar space. The process is patchy and individuals may have predominantly one or the other histological type. As the disease progresses fibrosis in the alveolar walls impairs gas transfer and disrupts the pulmonary vasculature; in addition there is collapse of small parts of the lung, leading to loss of functioning bronchoalveolar units. A 'loss of units pattern' is sometimes seen in mild cases, when lung restriction and loss of volume is accompanied by relative preservation of the corrected transfer factor (KCO). The histology of lung fibrosis in CFA and that seen with connective tissue diseases are similar.

There is an association of lung fibrosis with the organ-specific autoimmune diseases such as autoimmune thyroid disease and chronic active hepatitis.

Answer to questions 105–106

105 a) i) Right bundle branch block
    ii) Left axis deviation
    iii) First degree heart block.

b) Left axis deviation is commonly caused by left anterior hemifascicular block. The ventricular mass is depolarized from impulses generated at the sinoatrial node, and there is conduction delay to atrioventricular nodal depolarization. The left posterior hemifascicle is the only connection between the node and the ventricular mass.

c) Syncope is evidence of the intermittent failure of left posterior hemifascicle conduction and therefore complete atrioventricular block. This is an indication of permanent pacing.

106 a) This lady has presented with pulmonary hypertension and right-sided heart failure. Pulmonary hypertension rarely occurs independently and normally the symptoms and signs of the primary causative disease predominate. In the absence of other causes the differential diagnosis in a young female lies between **primary pulmonary hypertension** and **chronic pulmonary emboli.**

    Very small pulmonary emboli (microemboli) cause few or no symptoms. Repeated emboli over several months result in the development of pulmonary hypertension. A proportion of these cases are associated with pregnancy (usually following) or the oral contraceptive pill. Emboli from trophoblastic or breast tumours may rarely cause pulmonary hypertension. The diagnosis is made when asymmetric occlusions of pulmonary arteries can be demonstrated at angiography. Generally patients have an angiographic appearance identical to primary pulmonary hypertension; in such cases if no source of multiple emboli is apparent a diagnosis of primary pulmonary hypertension is made.

b) The essential investigation is cardiac catheterization, i) to confirm pulmonary hypertension and assess the right heart function; ii) to measure the wedge pressure and exclude mitral stenosis and other left heart causes of pulmonary hypertension; iii) by measuring the oxygen content to assess or exclude a significant right-to-left shunt; iv) to perform a pulmonary angiogram. Pulmonary angiography is rarely able to distinguish between microembolic disease and primary pulmonary hypertension.

    Definitive treatment of primary pulmonary hypertension is heart–lung transplantation. If detected early, microembolic disease may be treated by anticoagulation.

107 A

a) The blood gases are consistent with **chronic mild alveolar hypoventilation**, slightly reduced pO_2, a raised pCO_2, and a compensated respiratory acidosis. This lady is a typical 'Pickwickian'. This is the label given to patients with normal mechanical ventilatory function who underbreathe. There are three factors associated with the syndrome: i) obesity, ii) mild obstructive airways disease and smoking, and iii) reduced central drive to breathe, i.e. a reduced sensitivity to pCO_2.

Investigations include full pulmonary function tests, and sleep studies, i.e. monitoring of blood gases at night, since the degree of hypoventilation increases during sleep and apnoeic episodes may be observed.

b) Treatment is weight reduction, stopping smoking, and using nasal cannulae with compressed air at night to increase ventilation and reduce the number of apnoeic episodes. Long term complications of the syndrome include cor pulmonale and polycythaemia.

B

a) An elevated serum creatinine subsequent to the trimethoprim; the normal urea makes a more sinister explanation unlikely. Trimethoprim competes with creatinine for excretion by the distal convoluted tubule.

Disproportionate increase in serum urea/creatinine concentration

Urea > Creatinine	Creatinine > Urea
Dehydration/pre-renal failure	Liver disease
Gastrointestinal haemorrhage	Trimethoprim/Septrin
Acute-on-chronic renal failure	Rhabdomyolysis
Corticosteroids	Dialysis
Tetracyclines	Racial—Blacks
Infection	Pregnancy
Post surgery	Vomiting

108 a) Tuberculous meningitis or cryptococcal meningitis are the most likely diagnoses. Herpes simplex encephalomyelitis is less likely, given the normal MRI scan and low CSF glucose. A partially-treated bacterial meningitis might result in similar CSF findings.

b) Cryptococcus — Indian ink staining may demonstrate the presence of cryptococcal organisms in the CSF. Culture with special media (e.g. cyclohexamide-free agar or Saboraud's medium) may also be helpful to confirm the diagnosis. Direct detection of cryptococcal antigen in CSF is now available in many centres.

Tuberculosis — Ziehl–Nielsen or auramine staining for acid-fast bacilli and culture for tubercle bacilli should be set up. PCR-based tests for *M. tuberculosis* are now becoming more widely available, but specificity and sensitivity are still variable, and false positive results are common.

c) A treatment regimen to cover both cryptococcal and tuberculous meningitis should be started. Pending the results of specialist CSF investigations, it would be prudent to initiate therapy with a third generation cephalosporin and acyclovir, to cover a bacterial infection and HSV, which may present with a similar picture. Quadruple therapy for *M. tuberculosis* should include rifampicin, INH, pyrazinamide and ethambutol; intravenous amphotericin is the drug of choice for cryptococcal meningitis, though other anti-fungal agents (e.g. flucytosine) may be added.

Some authorities advocate the use of high dose steroids for patients with tuberculous meningitis. In this patient the baseline dose of prednisolone should at least be doubled to achieve the same immunosuppressive effect, as rifampicin is a potent enzyme-inducing agent.

109 A

a) At this stage she fulfils the criteria for a diagnosis of **benign paraproteinaemia**. These are:

1) A relatively low concentration of paraprotein (<20 g/l)
2) Absence of Bence–Jones protein
3) Absence of immune paresis
4) A normal skeletal survey
5) A normal percentage of plasma cells in the bone marrow (<4%); occasionally the percentage is greater than 4% but definitely less than 10%
6) Maintenance of a constant level of paraprotein over a period of time.

Benign paraproteinaemia may be found in the normal healthy adult population with a frequency of up to 1% and this increases to 3% in those over 70 years of age. It may also be found in hospitalized patients suffering from a wide range of non-lymphoproliferative disorders, e.g. liver disease, connective tissue disease and neoplasia of the gut and lung.

b) Regular outpatient follow-up is required to monitor the paraprotein levels and to ensure that a malignant paraprotein does not develop. Bone marrow, skeletal survey and Bence–Jones protein estimation should be repeated if there is suspicion of malignant transformation.

B

a) Cushing's syndrome due to ectopic ACTH production.
Ectopic ACTH production usually presents with the metabolic features of steroid excess. These are hypertension, diabetes, muscle weakness and a hypokalaemic metabolic alkalosis. In addition, marked pigmentation may occur.

b) i) Chest X-ray. Oat cell carcinoma of the bronchus is the likely source in a smoker. Other potential sites include pancreas, thymus, thyroid and breast or carcinoid tumours.
   ii) Plasma ACTH level. Typically, very high levels are associated with ectopic ACTH production (>200 ng/l) and accompany high plasma cortisol levels (>1000 nmol/l).

110 a) Multiple myeloma with a serum IgG paraprotein.
The diagnosis may be confirmed by i) examining the urine for the
presence of Bence–Jones protein, which is present in 66% of
cases, ii) bone marrow examination to show an increased
percentage of plasma cells (>10%), and iii) skeletal survey to
show osteolytic areas, which are present in 60% of cases.

b) i) Clinically the patient is nephrotic and this would account for
the oedema and exertional dyspnoea. Nephrotic syndrome
is a common consequence of renal amyloid. The diagnosis
may be confirmed by renal biopsy.

ii) In addition the ECG changes suggest the possibility of
cardiac amyloid. This typically produces a restrictive
cardiomyopathy — a common cause of death in these
patients. Cardiac amyloid often presents with oedema,
shortness of breath and angina. The echocardiographic
appearance is often diagnostic, with increased thickness of
right and left ventricular walls, decreased amplitude of wall
excursion and the characteristic 'granular sparkle'.
Endomyocardial biopsy confirms the diagnosis.

The clinical signs and symptoms of amyloid may precede the
diagnosis of an underlying immune dyscrasia. Systemic AL
amyloid may complicate any B-cell dyscrasia, e.g. multiple
myeloma, macroglobulinaemia, lymphoma and benign
monoclonal gammopathy. Overall AL amyloid complicates 15%
of cases of multiple myeloma. Other clinical features include
carpal tunnel syndrome (this patient complains of median nerve
compression), peripheral and autonomic neuropathy,
macroglossia, gut involvement with malabsorption/
haemorrhage/perforation, hepatomegaly, hyposplenism,
non-thrombocytopenic purpura, arthropathy and bleeding
diathesis — factor IX and X deficiency.

111 a) Churg–Strauss syndrome.

b) Churg–Strauss syndrome is a medium-vessel granulomatous vasculitis characterized by a triad of i) late onset asthma with or without allergic rhinitis, ii) a fluctuating eosinophilia, and iii) an extrapulmonary vasculitis involving two or more organs, e.g. the peripheral nervous system, skin, or kidney. The condition characteristically responds well to steroids.

c) i) Interstitial nephritis secondary to antibiotic therapy.
    ii) Cholesterol emboli — occur in arteriopaths and may be associated with an eosinophilia and occasionally a transiently low C3.

112 A

a) Inappropriate antidiuretic hormone secretion with hyponatraemia, hypouricaemia, and inappropriately high urinary sodium excretion and urinary (cf plasma) osmolality. The smoking history suggests the possibility of an underlying bronchial carcinoma.

b) Increased urate clearance — not a dilutional effect!

c) i) Establish and treat the underlying cause
    ii) Fluid restriction
    iii) Demethylchlortetracycline — antagonizes the effects of antidiuretic hormone secretion on the distal tubules.

Causes of true inappropriate antidiuretic hormone secretion include:

1) Malignancy — bronchial (small cell carcinoma), pancreas, lymphoma
2) CNS — head injury, meningitis, raised intracranial pressure, Guillain–Barré
3) Chest — infection, intermittent positive pressure ventilation
4) Drugs — chlorpropamide, cyclophosphamide, carbamazepine, vincristine, opiates, amitriptyline
5) Miscellaneous — acute intermittent porphyria, schizophrenia.

B

a) Measurement of plasma lipids. The patient has pseudohyponatraemia due to nephrotic syndrome and secondary hyperlipidaemia. The clues to this are: firstly the normal measured plasma osmolality (cf the calculated osmolaity of $2 \times ([Na^+] + [K^+]) + [Ur] + [Gl] = 254$), the low albumin and nephrotic range proteinuria.

Plasma sodium is measured in the aqueous phase and a false low reading is not uncommon in hyperlipidaemic states such as the nephrotic syndrome. More rarely, a raised serum protein, e.g. with a paraprotein, may give a milder pseudohyponatraemia.

Note: nephrotic syndrome is associated with raised levels of cholesterol (LDL) and when hypoalbuminaemia is severe, with elevated levels of triglyceride (VLDL). Chronic renal failure per se is associated with hypertriglyceridaemia.

113 a) There are two pacing spikes for each QRS complex: one precedes the P-wave and is therefore generated by an atrial pacing lead. The second precedes the QRS and is generated by a ventricular lead.

Atrial pacing will be inhibited by a native P-wave. Absence of native P-waves indicates sinus node disease.

If the AV node was functioning, the P-waves generated by the atrial pacing lead would cause a normal QRS complex. This does not happen, and in the absence of a normal QRS complex there is a paced beat (left bundle branch block morphology) — this indicates failure of atrioventricular conduction.

114 a) 400 mmol. Calculated from: 1/3 body weight (approx. vol of distribution) × base excess

b) Ethylene glycol poisoning. Recognized complications include cardiac failure and arrhythmias, pulmonary failure and acute renal failure which may complicate oxalate deposition.

c) i) Removal of ethylene glycol by haemodialysis; ii) treatment of acidosis; iii) ethanol infusion.

The causes of high anion gap acidosis are legion and include all causes of lactic acidosis. In the context of an overdose, consideration should be given to aspirin, paracetamol, methanol and ethylene glycol toxicity.

Ethylene glycol (antifreeze) is metabolized to oxalate, via glycoaldehyde and glycollate. The oxalate precipitates in the urine as calcium oxalate, causing crystalluria. Typically, it takes 12 hours from ingestion for symptoms to develop, somewhat less than is the case for methanol. Methanol toxicity is due to metabolism to the toxic metabolite formate and is dominated clinically by visual symptoms.

Optimum treatment, for both methanol and ethylene glycol toxicity, consists of bicarbonate dialysis to remove the toxin and treat the acidosis, and an ethanol infusion. Ethanol is preferentially metabolized by alcohol dehydrogenase, for which both methanol and ethylene glycol are substrates, thus preventing the generation of toxic metabolites.

115 a) Renal artery stenosis due to fibromuscular dysplasia.

b) The disease is bilateral — in unilateral disease, one would expect an increased renal vein renin from the affected kidney, with suppression of the unaffected kidney.

c) In a young woman fibromuscular dysplasia is the most likely cause. The treatment of choice is percutaneous angioplasty in this case. Atheromatous disease in older patients may require surgery.

d) Following renal artery angioplasty or surgical bypass, a considerable diuresis may occur. Careful monitoring and rehydration are needed, and the patient's antihypertensive therapy may require modification.

116 a) Multiple myeloma complicated by proximal renal tubular acidosis (type II). Investigations show a normochromic normocytic anaemia, an elevated ESR, hypercalcaemia, and an elevated alkaline phosphatase (note: alkaline phosphatase is only elevated when a pathological fracture occurs: the patient presents with back pain). The hyperchloraemic hypokalaemic metabolic acidosis and glycosuria in the presence of a normal plasma glucose are typical of proximal renal tubular acidosis. Other recognized features of proximal renal tubular acidosis include aminoaciduria, and increased urate and phosphate clearance with concomitant hypouricaemia and hypophosphataemia — the Fanconi syndrome.

In type II renal tubular acidosis, the proximal tubules fail in their normal function of reabsorption of bicarbonate (HCO_3^-) — normally approximately 85% of the filtered bicarbonate load. There is therefore an increased delivery of bicarbonate to the distal tubule, which is unable to reabsorb the excess, resulting in bicarbonaturia. As the serum bicarbonate falls, so does the proximal tubular bicarbonate concentration until it is below the T_{max} for bicarbonate, at which point bicarbonaturia ceases and net acid production and excretion are balanced. It is because of this that, unlike RTA type I, additional buffering from bone is not required and therefore osteomalacia and hypercalciuria do not occur. Sodium is the obligate cation lost with bicarbonate in the urine and the resulting volume depletion leads to stimulation of the renin–angiotensin–aldosterone pathway and hence to hypokalaemia. Hyperchloraemia is a result of eventual compensatory enhanced sodium and chloride reabsorption in response to hypovolaemia.

b) The appropriately low urine pH in this patient is explained by the fact that this was an early morning sample. Low urine flow at this time allows adequate acidification by a normal distal tubule.

c) i) To confirm the diagnosis of multiple myeloma: skeletal survey, bone marrow examination, measurement of serum immunoglobulins, protein electrophoresis and urine examination for Bence–Jones protein; ii) to confirm the diagnosis of proximal renal tubular acidosis: bicarbonate loading test. In a HCO_3^- loading test, the T_{max} for HCO_3^- (tubular maximal reabsorption of HCO_3^-) is soon exceeded and a fractional HCO_3^- excretion of greater than 15% of the filtered load occurs in cases of proximal renal tubular acidosis (compared with approximately 5% in distal renal tubular acidosis).

d) Albumin — amino acids and Bence–Jones proteins do not register on urinary dipsticks.

117 a) The most likely diagnosis is a **renal malignancy**. Thrombosis of veins occurs when the renal pelvis is involved. The left testicular vein joins the renal vein, while on the right it joins the inferior vena cava. A left varicocoele is strongly suggestive of renal pathology, and varicocoele is diagnosed in up to 10% of patients with renal carcinoma. The thrombus may stretch to the right atrium and cause right sided congestion. Renal carcinoma is a great 'mimic' and should be considered in all patients in this age group with a PUO. This patient did not present with the classic presentation of fever, a mass, haematuria and loin pain.

The patient has an erythrocytosis. Up to 40% of patients with renal adenocarcinoma are anaemic at presentation, but 4% have increased red cell production due to dysregulation of erythropoietin production.

b) Urine dipstick for blood and protein, and cytological examination of the urine are required. Special imaging is then indicated. Intravenous urography still has a place, but ultrasound has a sensitivity of 95%. CT scanning is better for staging renal carcinoma, and may define the extent of venous thrombosis.

118 a) The bicarbonate concentration is 14.5 mmol/l.

Anion gap = {[Na⁺] + [K⁺]} − {[Cl⁻] + [HCO₃⁻]}

Anion gap = $\{[Na^+] + [K^+]\} - \{[Cl^-] + [HCO_3^-]\}$

b) Renal tubular acidosis type I — the biochemical picture of a hyperchloraemic hypokalaemic acidosis with a normal anion gap is typical. The patient is unable to acidify the urine despite having a metabolic acidosis. Nephrocalcinosis and renal colic are well-recognized complications of distal renal tubule acidosis and account for the loin pain.

Note: An NH_4Cl loading test is only of use if the patient does not have a systemic acidosis. Conversely the patient does not have renal tubular acidosis if the pH of the urine is less than 5.5.

Distal and proximal renal tubular acidosis: causes

Distal renal tubular acidosis	Proximal renal tubular acidosis
Primary	Primary
Hereditary	Hereditary
Acquired	Wilson's disease
Autoimmune disease	Galactosaemia
Hypergammaglobulinaemia	Cystinosis
Sjögren's disease	Lowe's syndrome
Chronic active hepatitis	Fructose intolerance
Nephrocalcinosis	Autoimmune disease
Hyperparathyroidism	Sjögren's syndrome
Vitamin D intoxication	Dysproteinaemic states
Medullary sponge kidney	Multiple myeloma
Idiopathic hypercalciuria	Drugs
Tubulo-interstitial disease	Acetazolamide
Obstructive uropathy	Lead
Chronic pyelonephritis	Tetracyclines
Sickle cell disease	Miscellaneous
Drugs	Hypocalcaemia
Analgesic nephropathy	Hyperparathyroidism
Lithium	Amyloid
Amphotericin	Nephrotic syndrome

119 a) Epigastric discomfort; vomiting; nausea; sweating and hyperpyrexia; irritability, tinnitus, deafness, tremor; increased respiratory rate (pulmonary oedema); dehydration; hypokalaemia; bruising/purpura — secondary to hypoprothrombinaemia.

b) Both acid–base and fluid/electrolyte disturbances occur: initially, respiratory alkalosis; later, metabolic acidosis; hyper- or hypoglycaemia may occur.

c) Initial respiratory alkalosis is due to direct stimulation of the respiratory centre by salicylate. To compensate for this, bicarbonate is secreted in the urine, with loss of Na, K and water. The reduction in bicarbonate reduces the buffering capacity of blood.

Acidosis develops partly from the presence of salicylic acid, and partly as a result of interference with intermediary metabolism — e.g. TCA cycle inhibition results in an increase in lactate and pyruvate; stimulation of fat catabolism causes ketone body and β-hydroxybutyrate production (also starvation and dehydration); accelerated protein catabolism causes aminoacidaemia/uria.

Salicylates uncouple oxidative phosphorylation, thereby increasing oxygen utilization and carbon dioxide production; energy dissipated as heat and increased tissue glycolysis occurs. Severe dehydration can result, with pre-renal renal failure.

d) 300–500 mg/l at 6 hrs: mild toxicity
500–750 mg/l: moderate toxicity
>750 mg/l: severe toxicity
>1000 mg/l: consider haemoperfusion/dialysis.

e) i) Gastric aspiration/lavage — ipecacuanha in a child
ii) Activated charcoal orally
iii) Correction of dehydration with i.v. saline
iv) Correction of hypokalaemia
v) Correction of severe metabolic acidosis with i.v. bicarbonate
vi) Tepid sponging
vii) Forced alkaline diuresis if salicylate level >750 mg/l — monitor CVP. Urine pH 8–8.5
viii) Haemodialysis or haemoperfusion
ix) Vitamin K for hypoprothrombinaemia.

120 a) The patient presents with pyrexia, a right pleural effusion and leg oedema. Investigations reveal anaemia of chronic disease, an elevated ESR, hypoalbuminaemia, increased gammaglobulins, mildly deranged liver function tests and blood cultures positive for *Streptococcus milleri*. **The clinical picture is typical of an S. milleri hepatic abscess.**

Only 50% of patients complain of abdominal pain and a similar proportion have palpable hepatomegaly. Blood cultures are positive in 50–60% of cases and the organism is grown from aspirated pus in over 90% of cases.

The diagnosis should be confirmed by hepatic ultrasound, which has a sensitivity of over 90%.

Streptococcus milleri, a facultative anaerobe, accounts for over 80% of pyogenic hepatic abscesses in the UK. Sixty percent of cases are associated with underlying disease, e.g. cholangitis, appendicitis, diverticulitis, Crohn's disease, or carcinoma of the colon. The incidence is highest in males and occurs more commonly in diabetics and alcoholics.

b) Management in this case is straightforward and consists of drainage of the abscess, and antibiotics. In cases where blood cultures are negative, it is essential to exclude hydatid and amoebic causes of hepatic abscess (by the appropriate serological tests, stool examination and CT scan) prior to drainage. Drainage may be percutaneous or open. *Streptococcus milleri* is penicillin-sensitive and 2–6 weeks' therapy with a combination of penicillin and gentamicin is recommended.

121 a) Lateral medullary syndrome of Wallenberg.

b) Patients have dysphagia and dysarthria, ipsilateral cerebellar signs, ipsilateral Horner's syndrome, ipsilateral reduction in pinprick and temperature in the face, and contralateral pinprick and temperature loss in the limbs.

c) i) In the medulla (laterally placed)
ii) the posterior inferior cerebellar artery, though in 25% of cases the syndrome arises from vertebral artery occlusion.

d) Dysphagia/dysarthria — IXth and Xth nuclei. Vomiting — nucleus ambiguus; hiccough — reticular formation; vertigo — vestibular nuclei; cerebellar ataxia of the limbs on the side of the lesion — inferior cerebellar peduncle; Horner's syndrome — ipsilateral — descending autonomic fibres; reduced pinprick and temperature sensation on the face on the side of the lesion — Vth nucleus; reduced pinprick and temperature sensation over the opposite limbs — lateral lemniscus (the pain/temp fibres synapse in the posterior horn, and 2nd order neurons give rise to fibres that cross in the cord, joining the contralateral spinothalamic tract, which reaches the thalamus via the lemniscus lying in a *lateral* position in the pons and medulla).

122 a) Mesangiocapillary glomerulonephritis (MCGN) type II — dense deposit disease, associated with facial lipodystrophy.

Investigations show an active urine sediment and the principal clues to the diagnosis of MCGN II are the serological picture of a low C3 and normal C4 coupled with the registrar's description of the patient, which would be consistent with the appearance of facial lipodystrophy.

Measurement of serum C3 nephritic factor (C3NeF), an antibody which results in stabilization of the alternative pathway convertase, and complement consumption, is present in up to 70% of cases.

b) Common causes of renal impairment associated with a low C3 include:

1) Systemic lupus erythematosus
2) Idiopathic MCGN type II and III
3) Post-streptococcal nephritis
4) Infective endocarditis
5) Shunt nephritis.

The other possible disorders are less likely for a number of reasons, not least because they would all be expected to activate the classical complement pathway as well as the alternative pathway, and have low levels of C4 and total haemolytic complement.

There are no features to support a diagnosis of systemic lupus erythematosus, post-streptococcal nephritis or infectious endocarditis.

C3NeF is detected in 20–30% of cases of mesangiocapillary glomerulonephritis type I; there is however no association with facial lipodystrophy.

123 a) Wenckebach phenomenon: progressive second degree atrioventricular block.

There is progressive atrioventricular delay (P–R interval) until there is one period of complete atrioventricular block, after which the cycle restarts.

124 a) This is a nodal rhythm with clear retrograde P-wave conduction, notably in V1–V3.

125 a) Guillain–Barré syndrome.

b) Lumbar puncture:
   CSF Normal pressure
   Raised protein (N = 45 mg/dl)
   Normal cell numbers

   The differential diagnosis of a raised CSF protein and normal cell count and glucose level includes spinal cord block (Froin's syndrome); intracranial tumour (commonly internal acoustic neuroma).

c) Most patients are initially managed on a general ward by urinary catheter, nasogastric feeding, and physiotherapy. It is vital to keep joints mobile and functional; pressure area care, maintenance of morale/psychological state of both patient and family are important aspects of management.

   Spirometry and blood gases should be regularly monitored as rapid deterioration may require intensive care. Criteria for admission to ICU include i) severe weakness, ii) fall in vital capacity to <1.1 litres, and iii) infection and increasing hypoxia and hypercapnia. Ventilatory support, often with a tracheostomy, may be required for weeks or months.

   The role of immunosuppression/steroids is controversial, but plasma exchange may be beneficial.

   Prognosis in Guillain–Barré — patients avoiding ventilation often recover completely, and ventilated patients may have surprisingly little residual handicap, though long-term sequelae and the need for rehabilitation are commoner in this group. Less than 5% of patients have a recurrence of the disease.

d) Miller–Fisher syndrome — external ophthalmoplegia, ataxia, areflexia
   Polyneuritis cranialis — diffuse cranial nerve involvement
   Chronic relapsing polyneuritis.

126 a) Minimal change glomerulonephritis presenting with the nephrotic syndrome. Minimal change glomerulonephritis is most commonly idiopathic but may be associated with i) atropy, ii) drugs, e.g. aspirin and other non-steroidal anti-inflammatory agents, iii) lymphoproliferative disorders, and iv) viral infections.

b) The patient has developed renal vein thrombosis. Clinical clues to this are the deterioration in renal function, loin pain and haematuria. The history of acute shortness of breath suggests the possibility of secondary pulmonary embolism. There is a well-recognized increase in the incidence of venous thrombosis in nephrotic patients. Factors contributing to this increased risk include: i) loss of fibrinolytic factors in urine — principally antithrombin III but also protein C, protein S and plasminogen, ii) increased synthesis of clotting factors — factors V, VIII and fibrinogen, iii) thrombocytosis, and iv) over-diuresis, as in this case resulting in dehydration, reducing renal blood flow and increasing viscosity.

127 a) Acute renal failure and haemoptysis due to **antiglomerular basement membrane disease**. The differential diagnosis includes Wegener's granulomatosis, microscopic polyarteritis and systemic lupus erythematosus.

i) Is he a smoker? Is there any history of exposure to petrol, solvents/paints? These are recognized risk factors for lung haemorrhage in anti-GBM disease; other risk factors include recent infection and pulmonary oedema.

ii) Does he have any history of arthralgia, myalgia, rash, nasal symptoms, or jaundice? What has happened to his weight?

b) Urine microscopy evidence for an active urinary sediment; blood gases; group and save; anti-GBM assay; antineutrophil cytoplasmic antibody titre (ANCA) — elevated in cases of Wegener's granulomatosis and microscopic polyarteritis; antinuclear antibody titre (ANF); lung function tests — KCO is elevated with pulmonary haemorrhage; renal ultrasound and biopsy.

ECG changes are due to hyperkalaemia; CXR changes are due to lung haemorrhage or oedema.

c) Treatment of hyperkalaemia and fluid overload — intravenous calcium, dextrose/insulin, Ca resonium, acute dialysis. Acutely, plasma exchange is of benefit in removing the circulating anti-GBM antibody and is of particular benefit in the treatment of lung haemorrhage. This should be combined with immunosuppressive therapy in the form of high-dose corticosteroids and cyclophosphamide, the latter being replaced after 2 months with azathioprine. Overall survival is good but the renal prognosis in anti-GBM disease is poor as the diagnosis is often late.

128A

a) Chondrocalcinosis. The patient has **haemochromatosis**.
Haemochromatosis is an autosomal recessive inborn error of
metabolism which leads to a positive iron balance. Males are
affected more commonly than females and usually present in the
4th–6th decades.

The classic triad of i) diabetes, ii) hepatomegaly and iii) the
slate-grey skin pigment (due to increased melanin deposition)
may be accompanied by hypogonadotrophic hypogonadism,
chondrocalcinosis, dilated cardiomyopathy, weakness and weight
loss.

Note: There is an increased incidence of hepatoma in patients
with cirrhosis.

b) Measure serum iron and ferritin concentrations: both will be
elevated and serum transferrin saturation will be greater than
80%.
Measure blood glucose, which will be elevated.
Measure liver function tests.
Gonadotrophin and testosterone levels will be low.
Liver biopsy will show iron overload and the degree of hepatic
damage.
Desferrioxamine infusion will show increased urine iron
excretion.
X-ray the knees to show typical cartilage calcification.

B

a) The patient's elevated HbA1c confirms she is a **diabetic**
(HBA1c should be less than 6%).

b) Serum renin concentration is likely to be low.
The patient has impaired renal function, a hyperchloraemic,
hyperkalaemic metabolic acidosis, proteinuria and hypertension.
All these features are explicable by diabetic nephropathy and
Type IV renal tubular acidosis. Type IV renal tubular acidosis, or
hyporeninaemic hypoaldosteronism, is a well-recognized
complication of elderly, hypertensive, chronically hyperglycaemic
diabetics and is particularly likely to develop following
administration of prostaglandin synthetase inhibitors, suggesting
a causative role of prostaglandin deficiency in the generation of
this complication. Serum renin levels are low and result in
acquired hypoaldosteronism with resulting hyperkalaemia and
acidosis.

c) An arrhythmia due to the hyperkalaemia.

d) i) Hyperkalaemia per se, or ii) diabetic amyotrophy.

129 a) The history of increasing abdominal girth suggests ascites. The differential diagnosis of ascites includes: hepatic disease, nephrotic syndrome, protein losing enteropathy, right sided cardiac failure, and constrictive pericarditis, peritoneal infection (classically tuberculous), and disseminated peritoneal malignancy. The normal cardiac examination and lack of peripheral oedema would suggest either peritoneal infection or malignancy. In the absence of other signs of infection, the most likely diagnosis is **ovarian carcinoma**.

b) The ovarian malignancy should be confirmed by pelvic and trans-vaginal ultrasound examination, followed by CT scanning. The diagnosis may be confirmed by ascitic tap, followed by cytological examination, or at laparoscopy.

This woman was shown to have a genetic abnormality of both her BRCA1 and BRCA2 gene. BRCA1 (breast cancer associated gene) is associated with breast and ovarian cancer. Up to 85% of patients with mutations of this gene will develop breast cancer, while 60% will develop ovarian cancer. BRCA2 gene mutations are also associated with breast and ovarian cancer, but linkage is weaker than with the BRCA1 gene. These genes are examples of tumour suppressor genes and mutations predispose to malignancy. More than 200 mutations have been defined. Environmental and dietary factors also affect the probability of developing malignancy in the context of genetic abnormalities of this type.

130 a) The endoscopic examination should be completed. This patient is not necessarily bleeding from the varices and the gastric mucosa and duodenum should be visualized if technically feasible. This patient was found to have a large **duodenal ulcer**, which was oozing blood. There was no evidence that the varices were bleeding. In the emergency situation, injection of the ulcer with adrenaline and a sclerosant is indicated.

b) This patient requires resuscitation, ideally in a high dependency unit where he may be haemodynamically monitored. Further urgent blood samples for clotting studies and cross-matching should be sent. It is routine practice to commence intravenous H2 antagonists, but these have not been shown to decrease the frequency of rebleeding in this context.

Up to 50% of patients with demonstrable varices and GI bleeding are shown to be bleeding from another site. Full upper GI endoscopy is therefore mandatory. There is no place for prophylactic sclerotherapy, even in this patient with large varices, living in a remote area. Banding, sclerotherapy, intravenous vasopressin or octreotide are used in the emergency situation, for the treatment of variceal bleeding. Medical therapy with nitrates and beta blockers has been shown to be as effective in preventing mortality as banding or sclerotherapy. This patient is therefore a candidate for medical therapy.

131 (a) Functional C1 esterase inhibitor deficiency. Patients with C1 esterase deficiency are all heterozygotes and have one normally functioning allele. They typically present with angio-oedema in the absence of urticaria. In deficient patients the abnormal allele codes for the production of either no protein, or a defective protein. Antigenic testing in the latter case will be normal. The diagnosis of a functional deficiency is confirmed by doing a special functional assay performed on a citrated plasma sample. In cases of antigenic deficiency, the C1 esterase inhibitor level is often lower than 50% due to accelerated catabolism of the protein encoded by the normal allele in these heterozygous patients. The positive candida throat swab was probably due to previous antibiotic therapy.

b) Arrangements should be made for C1 esterase inhibitor concentrate to be available in Accident and Emergency for use on a named patient basis. Fresh frozen plasma may also be used if the above is not available. Adrenaline, antihistamines and hydrocortisone are of little use in acute attacks of angio-oedema in these patients.

c) The patient should be advised to inform her dentist of her problem, use a medic-alert bracelet, and to avoid ACE inhibitors. She should seek medical help early in the event of a severe upper respiratory tract infection, or the development of facial swelling, or pharyngeal discomfort. Where appropriate, family screening may be indicated.

132 a) This patient is most likely to have **extrahepatic obstructive jaundice secondary to a malignant process**. The two most likely possibilities are ampullary carcinoma and pancreatic carcinoma. Obstructive jaundice, with a microcytic anaemia, in a patient with underlying malignancy is more characteristic of ampullary carcinoma. Endoscopy with biopsy of the ampullary region is a method of making the diagnosis.

b) CT scan and ERCP are the radiological examinations with the highest yield in such patients. Abdominal ultrasound is less reliable, but will provide useful information, such as dilated extrahepatic bile ducts, or a mass in the pancreas or liver hilum.

133 a) Blood tests to determine K^+, urea, electrolytes, haemoglobin, platelets, white cell count and urgent blood film, clotting profile, fibrinogen and FDP levels. Urinalysis and culture. Blood and stool culture. Chest X-ray and 12 lead ECG.

b) This patient has **haemolytic uraemic syndrome**, caused by infection with enterotoxigenic *E. coli* O157: H7. Up to 6% of patients infected with this organism develop HUS. Infection follows ingestion of infected food such as beef, or unpasteurized milk. HUS is a recognized cause of microangiopathic haemolytic anaemia, which is characterized by fragmented red cells and thrombocytopenia. Importantly the clotting profile is typically normal or only mildly deranged.

c) The priority in this patient is the control of acute hyperkalaemia and acidosis. Intravenous insulin and dextrose should be administered. Calcium resonium, given orally or rectally, may be useful. Acute dialysis or haemofiltration may be required. A central line should be placed for monitoring of haemodynamic status, and careful monitoring of fluid balance is essential. Fresh frozen plasma is the mainstay of treatment for patients with HUS, and has been shown to improve outcome. Plasmapheresis may be required to provide intravascular space if the patient is oliguric.

The patient should undergo reverse barrier nursing. Stool culture of family and close contacts should be undertaken. The assistance of the hospital infectious control team should be sought. There is no role for antibiotic therapy, and anti-motility agents are contraindicated.

134 a) Eosinophilic fasciitis is by far the most likely cause. Causes of a systemic illness with hypereosinophilia include: drug reactions, lymphoma, aspergillosis, Lyme disease, filariasis and other parasitic infections, Churg–Strauss syndrome, eosinophilic fasciitis, eosinophilic myalgia syndrome, eosinophilic myositis, and eosinophilic leukaemia. The induration and swelling which this patient describes are typical of eosinophilic fasciitis. Scleroderma is not associated with eosinophilia, and the patient does not have sclerodactyly, nailfold vasculitis, or microstomia.

Blood film, biochemical profile, CPK and auto-antibody screen (including ANCA and antibodies to ENA), high resolution ultrasound or MR scan of an affected limb, CXR, ECG, echocardiogram, and full-thickness biopsy of muscle, skin and fascia should be performed. Nerve conduction studies and electromyography may be required, as the patient's neurological symptoms are likely to be due to compression of the median nerve.

b) It is important to elicit a history of any other foreign travel, particularly to Africa or Malaysia (filariasis). A history of exposure to drugs, toxins and other chemicals should be sought. Eosinophilic myositis is associated with exposure to L-tryptophan, and was a feature of the Spanish toxic oil syndrome.

135 a) You would look for evidence of a peripheral neuropathy, autonomic dysfunction, signs of rheumatoid vasculitis, signs of long-term steroid use: proximal myopathy, cataract, skin thinning, osteoporosis, psychosis.

b) Amyloidosis and **rheumatoid vasculitis**.

c) Urine microscopy, ESR, and CRP, blood count, blood glucose, full biochemical profile, 24-hour urine protein and creatinine clearance, rheumatoid factor and autoantibody screen, cryoglobulin measurement and complement levels, chest X-ray and ECG, SAP scan and/or rectal biopsy, renal ultrasound and biopsy.

d) Acute rheumatoid vasculitis may respond to immunosuppressive therapy with cyclophosphamide or plasma exchange. High dose steroids may be beneficial, but many of the features with which this patient presents are the consequence of previous and inappropriate steroid therapy. If a diagnosis of AA amyloidosis is confirmed, the prognosis is poor, but every attempt should be made to reduce the patient's acute phase response, and treat the fluid balance derangement secondary to her nephrotic syndrome.

136 a) The following tests are indicated: a differential white blood count and blood film, blood gases at rest and following exercise in order to assess whether the patient desaturates, departmental chest film with a lateral as well as PA, sputum culture and microscopy. After appropriate counselling an HIV test should be considered.

b) The most likely diagnosis is **pneumocystis pneumonia occurring in the context of HIV infection**. The X-rays of HIV positive patients with *Pneumocystis carinii* can demonstrate diffuse reticular infiltrates, consolidation of one or more lobes, or be normal in 10% of patients. Pleural effusion and pneumothorax have been reported. Immunodeficient patients are susceptible to a range of pulmonary infections, but it should not be forgotten that they also can present with 'conventional' organisms such as *S. pneumoniae* and *H. influenzae*. The co-presentation of pneumothorax and pneumocystis pneumonia in this context is well described. HIV infection may be associated with a low platelet count.

c) The patient should be admitted, and appropriate investigations performed to establish the cause of his infection. Sputum examination for pneumocystis may be useful, and induced sputum examination has a sensitivity of more than 80%. An induced sputum test should probably not be performed on this patient, as this could worsen his pneumothorax. Bronchoscopy may be required, and transbronchial biopsy or open lung biopsy is sometimes necessary. If the diagnosis of pneumocystis is confirmed, high dose co-trimoxazole should be given. His pneumothorax should be monitored and if it increases in size, aspiration or the insertion of a chest drain should be considered. This patient should receive prophylactic oral co-trimoxazole once his infection has cleared. Specialist referral to an HIV physician will be required to initiate treatment with an anti-retroviral therapeutic regime.

137 a) Parvovirus-associated arthropathy. Parvovirus
   arthropathy presents after a diarrhoeal illness which may be
   associated with a rash. Elevations of anticardiolipin and
   antiphospholipid antibodies are well described. The low positive
   rheumatoid factor is a coincidental finding.

   b) The main differential diagnoses are: i) a reactive arthritis
   following another viral infection (e.g. EBV, rubella, coxsackie), or
   a bacterial infection such as campylobacter or mycoplasma,
   or ii) the first presentation of a systemic inflammatory disease
   such as RA and SLE.

   c) Parvovirus serology (IgM) should be performed, which is
   diagnostic. Symptoms should resolve within 6 weeks. Many
   patients have anti-parvovirus IgG, which does not indicate an
   acute infection. This infection may be associated with a severe
   anaemia in some patients.

138 a) With loin pain, fever, confusion, and proteinuria, acute
   pyelonephritis should be considered first. However, this rarely
   causes renal failure. The most likely diagnosis in this particular
   patient is an **obstructive uropathy due to methysergide-
   induced retroperitoneal fibrosis**. Methysergide hydrogen
   maleate is a potent serotonin antagonist which was once widely
   used to treat migraine. It can cause both lung and retroperitoneal
   fibrosis.

   b) An urgent ultrasound will show bilateral pelvicalyceal
   obstruction.

   c) Percutaneous nephrostomy insertion and drainage (usually
   performed by a specialist radiologist) is the treatment of choice,
   in combination with a broad spectrum antibiotic. Hyperkalaemia,
   fluid overload or acidosis may require supportive measures.

   d) Cystoscopy and retrograde pyelography, or intravenous
   pyelography, will confirm the diagnosis. The ureters are typically
   drawn medially, and it should not be forgotten that pelvic
   malignancy is a common cause of obstruction in a female of this
   age. Other radiological investigations such as ovarian ultrasound,
   or CT scan of the abdomen, may need to be performed in this
   patient.

   e) Patients typically become polyuric after decompression of
   ureteric obstruction, and careful monitoring of fluid intake and
   output is essential. In some cases CVP monitoring may be
   required. Regular monitoring of serum electrolytes and
   bicarbonate is indicated. It is often useful to measure the
   electrolyte composition of the urine (patients may waste
   potassium in this situation) as this may help with the choice of an
   intravenous fluid repletion regime.

139 a) Hypertrophic obstructive cardiomyopathy, aortic stenosis or Wolff–Parkinson–White syndrome should be considered.

b) Subarachnoid haemorrhage due to an aneurysm or an A–V malformation may cause sudden death in young people.

c) The non-sedating anti-histamine terfenadine may predispose to arrhythmias, particularly torsades de points and ventricular fibrillation. Ketoconazole binds to slow-rectifying potassium channels in the cell in a similar way. Treatment with diuretics which reduce potassium, such as frusemide or thiazides, should not be given in patients on terfenadine. Terfenadine is now only available on prescription.

140 a) Appropriate investigations include: chest X-ray, blood gases, pulmonary function tests, high resolution CT scan of the chest with fine cuts through the lung bases. Fibreoptic bronchoscopy with transbronchial biopsy and bronchoalveolar lavage, or open lung biopsy, may be required to confirm a histological diagnosis of **inflammatory interstitial lung disease.**

In this patient chest X-ray demonstrated bilateral basal reticular infiltrates, confirmed on CT. Lung function tests demonstrated a severe restrictive disorder, and her vital capacity was 1.5 litres.

b) This woman had been treated for 10 years with daily nitrofurantoin and has developed interstitial lung fibrosis. Other drugs which can produce this include: 1) bleomycin and mitomycin; 2) cyclophosphamide, busulfan, melphelan; 3) lomustine, chlorozotocin; 4) phenytoin, carbamazepine; 5) amiodarone, lignocaine; 6) heroin, methadone; 7) aspirin or non-steroidal anti-inflammatory drugs; 8) gold, methotrexate and penicillamine; 9) procarbazine, colchicine; 10) high dose oxygen.

c) Lung fibrosis in this situation is unfortunately irreversible, and lung function often deteriorates despite stopping medication, with the development of pulmonary hypertension. She may be a candidate for lung or heart/lung transplantation.

141 a) This patient has **obstructive jaundice due to massive hepatobiliary ascariasis**. These symptoms would also be consistent with the diagnosis of gallstone obstruction of the common bile duct. The eosinophilia suggests a parasitic infection, but may be coincidental in a patient from this part of the world.

b) Repeat liver function tests and full blood count will be required. An abdominal ultrasound is indicated, to look for bile duct dilatation, the presence of gallstones or other intra- or extra-luminal pathology. Experienced ultrasound operators can confidently make the diagnosis of biliary ascariasis. ERCP is the definitive diagnostic examination and may demonstrate *Ascaris lumbricoides* worms protruding from the bile duct papilla.

c) Oral therapy with albendazole, mebendazole, pyrantel embonate or piperazine is effective for gastrointestinal infestation of *A. lumbricoides*. Bio-availability of these drugs in the biliary tract is not good, and intra-biliary infusion of vermicidal agents may be necessary. Follow-up ultrasound or ERCP must be performed to confirm disappearance of worms.

142 a) This patient has **lead poisoning**, due to the presence of this heavy metal in the drugs he has been taking for his joint pains. Such 'alternative' remedies, such as 'Ayurvedic' treatments, frequently contain heavy metals such as arsenic, lead or mercury, or other toxins. Their prescription and formulation are not, of course, regulated in the same way as conventional Western drugs.

Clinical features of lead poisoning include: peripheral motor neuropathy (particularly affecting the radial nerve), raised intracranial pressure and papilloedema, mood disturbance and memory impairment, alteration in bowel habit, typically constipation, abdominal pain, sideroblastic anaemia with basophilic stippling, blue lines around the gums, and proximal renal tubular acidosis.

b) Abdominal X-ray (tablets may be radio-dense and visible within the gut), examination of a blood film, and measurement of blood lead levels and delta-aminolaevulinic acid may all be informative in this patient. Nerve conduction studies may be helpful. Blood levels of lead: in children levels of more than 40 mg/dl, and in adults more than 50 mg/dl, are abnormally high.

Other 'medical' causes for abdominal pain include: diabetes mellitus, pre-eruptive phase of Herpes zoster, diphtheria, porphyria (particularly acute intermittent porphyria and variegate porphyria), syphilis, pneumonia or pulmonary embolus, sickle crisis, mesenteric angina, hereditary angio-oedema and Familial Mediterranean Fever (FMF).

c) Cessation of the patient's poisonous 'alternative' drug treatment is required. Chelation with EDTA or dimercaprol (BAL) may be required in acute lead poisoning.

143 a) The patient has a **primarily axonal neuropathy**, characterized by diminution of the action potential with normal conduction velocity.

Isoniazid, administered as part of the patient's anti-tuberculous chemotherapy regime, is the most likely cause.

b) Other causes of an axonal neuropathy include:
Hereditary Sensorimotor Neuropathy Type II (HMSN)
Diabetes
B_{12}-deficiency
Folic acid deficiency
Renal failure
Malignancy
Drugs — e.g. vinca alkaloids.

144 a) The patient has developed an **acute bacterial pneumonia** and is markedly leukopenic. The most likely explanation is that he has been prescribed allopurinol for his gout. This is a xanthine oxidase inhibitor and has resulted in the development of azathioprine toxicity leading to bone marrow suppression, leukopenia and acute sepsis.

Xanthine oxidase is one of a number of hepatic enzymes involved in the metabolism of azathioprine. In the normal population there is variation in the ability of individuals to metabolize this drug. Azathioprine should therefore be used cautiously, starting at a low dose, and with regular initial monitoring (within 1 week or less) of the full blood count and biochemical profile.

b) Emergency therapy of the patient's pneumonia is needed, with hydration, oxygen, bronchodilators and broad spectrum antibiotics. Allopurinol should be stopped, and acutely it would be advisable to stop the azathioprine. A specialist renal opinion should be sought about the optimal immunosuppressive regime which should be employed in the longer term. Colony stimulating factors may be useful in drug-induced leukopenia in patients whose marrow is slow to recover and who have life-threatening sepsis.

145 a) This patient is most likely to have **McArdle's disease**. McArdle's disease is a glycogen storage disease due to a genetic deficiency of muscle phosphorylase. This condition may remain unrecognized until early adulthood, frequently presents with painful muscle cramps after exercise, and affected patients are not infrequently labelled as having a functional disorder, or 'chronic fatigue' syndrome. Inheritance is autosomal recessive.

b) No rise in venous blood lactate is detected on exertion in these patients, and diagnosis is made by muscle biopsy, in which there is an elevated concentration in glycogen (which is structurally normal), and a deficiency in muscle phosphorylase.

146 a) Pulmonary hypertension is the most likely diagnosis. This may often present insidiously in the manner illustrated, and exertional breathlessness, tachypnoea, and effort syncope are classical features. In this patient, the use of an anorectic agent may be implicated. There is 'previous history' of obesity, but the patient's weight and height do not suggest that she is overweight at the time of the current presentation.

b) A detailed drug history is therefore required. It is becoming increasingly clear that there is an association between the use of anorectic drugs such as dexfenfluramine (Adifax) and the development of pulmonary hypertension. Many thousands of patients have used this type of drug, which may be obtained by conventional means or through 'specialist slimming clinics', and pulmonary hypertension is a rare, but increasingly well-defined, association of their use. The relevant medicolegal issues remain unresolved.

A history of pre-existing cardiac disease, other chronic chest disorders, previous thromboembolic disease, or an underlying systemic rheumatic condition (e.g. systemic sclerosis, rheumatoid arthritis) should also be sought.

c) The main investigations required are a full blood count, biochemical profile, blood gases, pulmonary function tests, ECG, CXR (and chest CT), and echocardiogram. A ventilation/perfusion scan, auto-antibody testing and cardiac catheterization may be indicated, depending on the clinical context and the severity of the condition.

147 a) The likely diagnosis is **Familial Benign Hypocalciuric Hypercalcaemia** (FBHH). Elevated serum calcium (sometimes >3.5 mmol/l), normal or slightly low phosphate, and borderline hypermagnesaemia (0.95–1.10 mmol/l) are typical. Three-quarters of patients have a 24-hour urinary Ca excretion of less than 2.5 mmol, which is clearly inappropriate in the context of serum *hyper*calcaemia. A patient with primary hyperparathyroidism would be expected to have an elevated urinary calcium excretion.

b) Evaluation of the ratio between urinary calcium clearance and creatinine clearance can help to distinguish between FBHH and primary hyperparathyroidism. In the former >80% subjects have a CaCl/CrCl ratio of <0.01. The majority of patients with primary hyperparathyroidism have values which are higher. A serum PTH should be measured. This is normal or mildly elevated in FBHH. Vitamin D levels are usually normal.

c) It has been estimated that up to 10% of patients who undergo 'successful' parathyroid surgery have FBHH, and patients should be warned about inappropriate surgery. A low calcium diet is not indicated, and management is generally conservative. Many patients with FBHH have been shown to have specific heterozygous mutations in the calcium-sensing receptor gene (often encoding defects in the extracellular part of the receptor). These mutations may result in an elevation of the threshold for calcium ion-responsive PTH release, and enhance the degree of calcium resorption within the kidney at a given blood calcium level. Some patients have other mutations, and genetic analysis is complex. If a kindred with FBHH is identified, referral to a specialist centre is indicated.

148 a) A history of foreign travel, injections, drug use/abuse, or similar previous episodes should be sought.

b) Investigations required are: blood cultures; blood film and clotting profile; throat swab; CPK, urinalysis, then proceeding to imaging of the painful area — US/CT.

c) Fluids and i.v. antibiotics — including cover for anaerobes — are indicated acutely. Consideration should be given to radiological and/or surgical drainage.

d) The most likely diagnosis is a local pyogenic infection/pyomyositis. Lemierre's syndrome — a metastatic infection due to systemic anaerobic infection caused by *Fusobacterium necrophorum* — was the diagnosis in this patient.

e) Historically, the condition was universally fatal, but with modern antibiotic regimes, radiological or surgical drainage, and other supportive therapy, most patients now survive, but prolonged hospital admission, with considerable morbidity, is common.

INDEX

NB: Numbers in the index refer to
questions not pages. Numbers in
italics indicate that specific mention
of the subject is made only in the
Answers section.